Walking
the
Night Road

Coming of Age in Grief

∽

ALEXANDRA BUTLER

Columbia University Press
New York

Columbia University Press
Publishers Since 1893
New York   Chichester, West Sussex
cup.columbia.edu
Copyright © 2015 Alexandra Butler
All rights reserved

A translation of C. P. Cavafy's poem "The God Abandons Antony" is reprinted
here by permission of Princeton University Press from *C. P. Cavafy:
Collected Poems*, edited by George Savidis, translated by Edmund Keeley
and Philip Sherrard (Princeton, N.J.: Princeton University Press, 1992).

Library of Congress Cataloging-in-Publication Data
Butler, Alexandra.
Walking the night road : coming of age in grief / Alexandra Butler.
         pages   cm
ISBN 978-0-231-16752-9 (cloth : acid-free paper)—ISBN 978-0-231-16753-6
(paperback : acid-free paper)—ISBN 978-0-231-53679-0 (e-book)
1. Butler, Alexandra—Family.   2. Lewis, Myrna I.—Health.   3. Glioblastoma
multiforme—Patients—Family relationships.   4. Glioblastoma multiforme—
Patients—United States—Biography.   5. Mothers and daughters—United
States.   6. Butler, Robert N., 1927–2010.   7. Women caregivers—United States—
Biography.   8. Caregivers—Psychology—Case studies.   9. Terminal care—
Psychological aspects—Case studies.   10. Grief—Case studies.   I. Title.

RC280.B7B88 2015
362.196994810092—dc23
2014045641

Cover design: Jordan Wannemacher
Cover image: © Ketuta Alexi-Meskhishvili

References to Web sites (URLs) were accurate at the time of writing.
Neither the author nor Columbia University Press is responsible for URLs
that may have expired or changed since the manuscript was prepared.

For Robin and Kon

When suddenly, at midnight, you hear
an invisible procession going by
with exquisite music, voices,
don't mourn your luck that's failing now,
work gone wrong, your plans
all proving deceptive—don't mourn them uselessly.
As one long prepared, and graced with courage,
say goodbye to her, the Alexandria that is leaving.
Above all, don't fool yourself, don't say
it was a dream, your ears deceived you:
don't degrade yourself with empty hopes like these.
As one long prepared, and graced with courage,
as is right for you who proved worthy of this kind of city,
go firmly to the window
and listen with deep emotion, but not
with the whining, the pleas of a coward;
listen—your final delectation—to the voices,
to the exquisite music of that strange procession,
and say goodbye to her, to the Alexandria you are losing.

—C. P. Cavafy, "The God Abandons Antony"

Acknowledgments

I WANT TO THANK MY GUARDIAN ANGEL JUDITH
Estrine, the first person after my father to read the manuscript of this book, and Helen Rehr, who is the reason it
is published. Jennifer Perillo of Columbia University Press is
a fantastic editor and a joy to work with, and Stephen Wesley,
Meredith Howard, Kathryn Jorge, Anne McCoy, and Jordan
Wannemacher all helped make transforming my manuscript
into a book possible.

Dan Blank, Lynne Griffin, Anna Goldstein, Anne
Burack-Weiss, Andrew Achenbaum, Tracy Brown, Jeanette
Takamura, Ursula Staudinger, Helen Rehr, Thomasena
Wilson, Morriseen Barrimore, Diane Meier, Barbara Paris,
Andrea Longacre-White, Brendan Fowler, Janelle Cori,
Beverly Torres, Caitlin Rider, Lina Mati, Anicka Yi, Ketuta
Alexi-Meskhishvili, Lisa Farjam, Mirabelle Marden, Sahra
Motalebi, Tina Tyrell, Cristina Bloom, Vicky Usle, Emily
Straight, Caitlin Wall, Eli Robinson, Isabel Penzlien, Alec
Coiro, Daniel Holzman, Karyn Starr, Will Reiser, Alex
Maynard, David Maynard, Dori Maynard, Marc Clopton,
Joan Retallack, Vicki Levy, Alexandra Sacks, Anna Kelly,
Marina Auerbach, Michael Trubkovich, Lev Trubkovich,
Maya Levin, and Katie Rudik all deserve my gratitude, as do
my big, beautiful Minnesota family and the intrepid Anne
Carlson.

I also want to thank Myrna Lewis, Robert Butler, Easter Schattner, Liz Hill, and Emil Eickhoff for nothing less than a wonderful childhood. My sister Carole Hall, my brothers-in-law Rick Guest, Jim Gleason, and Boots Hall, and my six nephews and nieces—B. J. Hall, Bobby Hall, Chooch Guest, Charlie Guest, Lauren Gleason, and Brendan Gleason—are all my best friends each in their own way. Marine Metreveli, with all her love and beauty, is a ballast of my life.

To two great authors and editors—who also happen to be my aunt and uncle—Diane Eickhoff and Aaron Barnhardt: thank you for your input, your support, and your dedication to this book and to this writer.

Cynthia and Christine Butler—you are more than sisters, sometimes mothers, sometimes friends. Sometimes I drive you crazy. (It's mutual.) Our relationship is hard to define but, as Cindy once said, the greatest part of it is love.

Finally, I want to thank my husband Kon Trubkovich, who showed me the toil and guts it takes to be an artist and who is the perfect mix of safety and adventure. And lastly to Robin Trubkovich, my gentle, focused, and kind one-year-old so intent on climbing stairs: You never seem to question you will reach the top. You are laughing all the way. Keep going, my love.

Walking the Night Road

YOU CAME INTO THE KITCHEN THAT NIGHT with only a T-shirt and no underwear. I was sitting with a friend in the living room as you went by. I could hear you breathing. You went foraging in the pantry. You knocked the cans and other objects off the shelf. You found a cereal box, pulled it out, and held it wrong side down, leaving a trail as you walked from the kitchen.

In the hallway you saw us. You saw my friend, and in your T-shirt and no underwear, you didn't stammer or apologize. There was no pause. But I remember your eyes as you passed.

I think about you at the doorway where you stood. I think about you in the dark house. I cross the house at night. I hear the floorboards creak and shift and recognize the weight of your footsteps in mine. I swim down—down in search of surface while the people come and go.

In daylight I make my way from the bed to sink, to street, to train, and back to bed again. And each day happens. I pass the places in the house where you fell. There is the bloodstain on your bedroom floor that only I can see. I know how to lean way down and find it crusting on the dark wood.

In the May that I was twenty-four, I had a presentiment of something coming for me. I had felt it all the year before. My mother and father went to England in May, for several weeks, and I stayed alone in their apartment.

I was one year out of Hampshire College, working at a place called Shadow Studios in Chelsea. I had studied film and video at school and rented the equipment for my final thesis there. One day I started chatting with the owner and he offered me a job at the front desk. I spent a year there, taking freelance jobs on TV shows and films that came through the studio.

Each day I rode my bike to work and back again, then out for the night, pedaling home in early morning, Uptown, along the Hudson. Sometimes I would sit and bring up the sun at the water's edge of West Fifty-fourth Street where weeping willows hang over reeds and water rocks. I fell asleep there once with my bike propped up and unchained, exhausted from the drunken peddling.

I felt more invincible, more at ease that summer than at any other time in my life. I somehow felt aware that it was a carefree time and soon it would be ending. Maybe that is a normal state of mind when a person is fresh out of college. And maybe it is normal for someone who has parents who are older. My mother had me when she was forty-two. I was her first child and the fifth child of my father, who was nearly fifty-three when I was born. Now she was sixty-five and he, seventy-six.

Life is slowly standing up knowing all the while you will go down. All I know is that when I was twenty-four, I was waking up fast, feeling the force of something approaching—a gathering of water, a gathering of waves.

I remember the day, carrying my bike up the stairs because the elevator had broken down, and she was sitting at the table in the kitchen when I came in. The window just behind her held the setting sun above the alley. The light was eating up the kitchen entirely. I held my fingers to my eyes to see her shape in all that whiteness and walked toward my mother's silhouette. It was the beginning of July.

She was rabid. She had called me several times from England over the past week, and I hadn't answered. She began to yell, banging her fists on the table.

Just leave!

I carried my bicycle down the stairs. I didn't return until I thought she was asleep, and when I lay down and closed my eyes, she came into my room and kissed my head, and we didn't speak of it again that night.

My mother did not get angry—not really. Sadness was her thing. When she felt anger she would crouch at the site of it and weep. Anger frightened her. She thought it was unnatural and dangerous, that it would lead to loss.

All my life it took only an apology, a show of kindness on my part, for her to forgive anything I did, and that is why I should have known right away that the woman in the light was not my mother.

A year always ends with December's succession to January. This time the coming year messed it all up. It jerked back and crashed into July, came down like an axe into summer, ending the life I had known and starting another.

My mother, Myrna Lewis, was a farm kid from southeastern Minnesota. She was proud of this. Only in the past few years have I come to see her as a lonely woman, someone who had many friends and hid herself from all of them. She was moody. Her mood could run the gamut from sorrow to elation; in an hour, she could go from lost to found. I had her memorized. I would begin to soothe before the darkness started.

She had struggled to build a life apart, and in many ways contrary to her family. And yet much of her life was focused on gaining their approval, which never seemed to come. She lived in fear that they would discover she had given up her Lutheran faith and they would disown her. She was particularly frightened that she could lose her mother.

We went home to Minnesota twice a year. She would brush my hair compulsively. She pulled me out of children's games to retie the ribbons of my dress. By four or five years old I had been trained to report that I worshipped Jesus Christ when I did not.

In New York City I was being raised atheist in a recoded spiritual environment. My parents' lives were focused around service. He was a doctor, she a social worker. They were stewards of nature, worshippers of animals, older people—children. They were generous with money and apart from travel, spare in their own lives. Their life was like a wordless hymn to a nameless god they would sooner dismiss than admit that they believed in. In my house religion was a bad word.

My father would get angry with her in Minnesota. He felt it was abusive to force a child to lie. Then she would collapse, dissolve into spineless flesh before us, traumatized and terrorized that she could lose them all. And I would step between her and my father, toy sized and furious as a guard dog. His arms would pull us both toward him. He gave up.

Of course I did not know that he was right. I was a child who did not know I was a child. My mother treated me as something else. She was a wonderful mother. Yet she was also a motherless child. I think I understand more what it is to be a twin than what it is to be another woman's daughter.

When I was five, I made the gaffe. I told one of my cousins I did not believe in angels. I did not know angels were a Christian thing. I thought that they were Disney characters, Tinker Bell or Merryweather.

My mother paced back and forth, got down on her knees, and took me by the shoulders. She made for me a trail of words to follow my way back, beneath the high arched eyebrows of her family.

All the photos of my grandmother Irene and I were taken in the first weeks of my life. She came to stay just after I was born and kept me in her room, waking my mother when I needed to be fed.

My mother always said Irene was wonderful with babies. She knew just how to hold them, and to impart so much through simple touch. And yet when my mother turned six, something came between them. She started to refuse her mother's lap. Irene told her that she was a bad child—so bad that she would be the death of her. She told my mom to pray to Jesus Christ or she would burn in hell. To my mother it felt as if Irene had begun to take her to the edge of the universe and hold her there to stare into the fall. That was when my mom started to avoid the house and help her father in the fields.

The break that occurred between these women never mended, and I think my mother divided in two. Half of her knew the peace of having been well loved. The other half I think was nearly destroyed.

I think my mother lived out the rest of her life as two separate women. Each one controlled a hand working over the same patch of life. One hand drew the world in a beautiful line and the other one erased it.

If you asked my mother's older brothers about Irene, they would describe a sweet and gentle woman, a pillar in the community, a devout Christian, the person who could be counted on to help when there was a fire, a tornado, a tragic death. In that respect, my mother followed in Irene's footsteps. And yet that common need or desire to help others did not mean they saw eye to eye on too much else. There was a dark side to Irene that somehow only her daughters knew. Irene would "get the blues," as she called it, and take to her bed in the middle of the day. Her daughters would try to cheer her up, to no avail.

When Irene was six years old, she had found her father hanging in the barn. She had gone to call him in for dinner, but she had played along the way. When they cut him down, he was still alive, but he died shortly after. Because her father had committed the mortal sin of suicide with no chance to repent, Irene believed he had gone to hell. She prayed that maybe he had repented in the final agonizing seconds of his life, but this she could never know for sure. She lived her life believing that if she had gotten there just a moment sooner, he could have been spared. The church refused to give him a place in hallowed ground. He was buried in a potter's field, and never discussed in the family. At school the children taunted Irene that he was in hell.

My mother came home from her first semester at college, having taken a class in psychology 101. She asked Irene if she blamed herself for her father's death. *How did you know?* Irene asked.

They found the potter's field in Mankato, Minnesota, but they never found where Christian Biel was buried. He was laid in an unmarked grave. They sat quietly in the cemetery. My mother hoped it gave Irene some peace. Perhaps it did, but by that time my mom was pulling away from her roots more than ever, and their relationship was showing new signs of strain.

My mother began to feel that something was wrong with her and that nothing she did could ever fully please Irene. My mother was the kind of daughter most mothers would have been bursting with pride over, first in her class. She was well liked by everyone. She was superneat. And even before she left home, she began to collect honors and scholarships as she had once collected gopher tails. But she felt like she was always walking on eggshells when she was around Irene. She never knew what might trigger an emotional outburst that would send Irene out of the room in the middle of a conversation or cause her to fall into a depression. This was especially true when it came to religion, the question of church attendance and Irene's suspicion that my mother had "lost her faith."

My mother learned to be cautious. To avoid discussions on sensitive topics and to divert discussions that were heading in a bad direction. This was a heavy price to pay to maintain a relationship, but my mother paid it again and again, knowing that if she ever came out with what she really wanted to say, it might be over between them.

I was six when Irene died, and I didn't cry because she was a stranger. She belonged to her other grandchildren. I had understood this very young. She was never cold yet always far away, respectful that the invisible line between her and my mother extended to me. A phone call came in the middle of the night, and my mother pulled me out of bed and carried me over to the window. We sang "Moon Over Alabama" until it was light.

When we went home to Minnesota, I waited at the cemetery gate in my new patent leather shoes. My mother crouched down by Irene's grave, and then she took me walking. Her father was just beyond town, looking over a field with her brother. When she spotted him, she dusted off my shoes, hoisted me on her shoulders, and walked toward my grandpa's silhouette.

I look at old photographs and try to imagine what my mom was like as a child. I can see her kicking up dirt on the country roads. She has dark eyes, sharp cheekbones, and a gap between her two front teeth. She has scratches on her brown legs and her socks are at her ankles. In one black-and-white photo she has black, lace-up shoes, and in another she is wearing an apron dress that has a round baby doll collar, brass buttons, and is cinched tight at her tiny waist.

It's hard to find anyone who is truly free. Most of us have someone with whom we are psychically ensnared. Someone whom we build ourselves so high to get away from; with whom we do battle for the meaning of all things. For Myrna this person was Irene. And it's Myrna for me.

Many generations can get caught up on one thing, one event that echoes down the line. My grandmother, my mother, and myself—we were strung up. All on Irene's father's noose from years before—like brainless pearls.

When I was little I thought that Minnesota was a snow globe, a real snow globe, with a bottom and glass sides. There is no place that I have been where the sky seems so round. It sits like a half globe on the land, as if it were fastened at its edges to the cornfield like a tent you can lift up to crawl under and escape.

A few days after my mom came home from England, she went to a party. It was thunder and lightning outside. Through my window, New York had been smudged. All the lights from the buildings on the East Side were strung up in the trees, like summer Christmas. It was July eleventh. My mother would recount this night often over the next sixteen months.

She had felt strange since returning from England, but she and my father had decided it was jet lag. She went to a friend's house for a dinner party and had a glass of wine. She was a notorious lightweight at drinking, and it wasn't completely odd that she became tipsy. Yet she was especially tipsy that night, and her host offered to walk her home. She laughed that it wasn't necessary.

She walked out of the building to the street, and in a moment she was lost. She had lived in this neighborhood for twenty-two years, and yet she couldn't find her way, though she was four blocks from her home.

She stopped several times to ask for directions but kept forgetting. Then all at once cars were screeching to a halt around her, and a stranger, grabbing her arm, pulled her from the street. She said the car lights seemed magnified, their details blurred. And the buildings lay bathed in puddles on the pavement. There were so many objects without names around her, so many thoughts and so few words that she could find to describe what was happening. The furrowed brows of countless strangers' faces filled with questions. She tried to say where she lived several times before she could find the right combination of words and numbers. Like picking a lock, desperation finally snapped the bolt of memory into place one last time. Never again would she go out alone. I think of her when it rains.

At sixty-five my mother looked ten years younger than her age. She had recently received her Ph.D. from Columbia in social work. She split her time between working at Mount Sinai Hospital School of Medicine and in her own private psychotherapy practice. Her specialty was male CEOs.

She had coauthored two books with my father, Robert Butler, a geriatrician and gerontologist. Their first collaboration, *Aging and Mental Health*, was published in 1973. It was the first comprehensive textbook ever published on the psychosocial aspects of older adulthood. It influenced a generation of practitioners in the field of aging.

Their second book, *Love and Sex After Sixty*, was published in 1976. It became an instant best seller. It challenged the ageist view that older adults could not or perhaps should not be having sex.

Several copies of this book were stacked in the corner of our living room and my schoolmates found them. From that moment, my parents were known among my friends as the "sexologists." I grew up trying not to watch my parents on TV discuss orgasms or age-related erectile dysfunction with Charlie Rose or Phil Donahue.

In her solo work my mother challenged the women's movement, through writing and lecturing, to address the issues of older women. She also supported younger women—particularly international students at Columbia University. She took a special interest in students who had come from eastern Europe. Often these girls were the first generation in their families to attend college. She offered herself to them as a mentor and a friend, hosting frequent dinners at our house. At the time I did not make the connection, but she had also been the first in her family to reach college.

My mother spoke sometimes of her old age, even of widowhood. She worried that my dad was getting old. She created a therapy group, which she named the Women's Longevity Group, where older women could meet to discuss issues like widowhood, dating, late-life career change, finance, health, and so on. She planned to facilitate the group starting in the coming fall.

My mother had always been a nerd, in many ways a loner. Books were her closest friends, and she always had a litany of hobbies. Now she was teaching herself to play blues harmonica from a book creatively titled *Blues Harmonica*. My mother was an obsessive autodidact with a bookcase dedicated solely to instructional books on seemingly every topic, from trading stocks to urban gardening.

One of my favorite stories is of her at sixteen trying to teach herself, from a book, how to swim. She was going to be a camp counselor and it was her plan to impress. My mother lay on a chair for days perfecting her stroke. That summer on the first day of camp she dove into a lake and immediately sank down to the bottom. Another counselor had to save her life.

After the night of the party, *Blues Harmonica* lay open for several weeks until I finally closed it in October.

When I woke on July twelfth, she had left the house. A pair of her shoes lay in the middle of the hallway just outside where our bedrooms met. I stepped over them on my way to the kitchen without giving it much thought. But that wasn't like her.

That morning seems so exaggerated now when I look back, and so supremely, so ridiculously, luxurious. I'm sipping coffee with my feet stacked up on the kitchen chair. I'm staring out into the alley, unaware that I'm having breakfast at the edge of my life. Within minutes all will change—had already months before. I think of that day, and everything about me seems slow, as if I am taking longer, storing up all that is lazy, freedom, safety, family.

Count back from ten. That is what the doctor once told me since I had trouble breathing when I thought of her. *Count back from ten.* As if that would help me. *Count back from ten* is not a way to find breath but a way to tell a story. A story such as this can be told only once it is done, and breathlessness subsides. *Count back from ten.* I go back to that day in my mind, and I can change it. I notice her shoes in the center of the hall, and the house pulls itself into focus. I can see how it truly was that day—all the things I didn't notice.

The house looked as if she'd brushed it over with a hurried hand. Things were open—drawers, cans, and closets. A pile of newspapers fanned out across the floor by the front door, and still I did not wonder. She must have dropped them as she ran, I thought. My mother was often late. But had I stopped to look, I would have seen the fear in the way the house had settled—a footstool that lay on its side, several books that had fallen from their shelves. When you count back, you can see a story from the end. I like that—the seemingly natural narrative that forms this way. With the end in my hand, the story becomes mine. I can have it all make sense, or I can lose my mind like she lost hers—like I lost her. But I can have my story.

I remember my cell phone ringing when I stepped out of the shower. I walked so leisurely toward it. I saw her number flashing, and almost let it go. I thought she probably wanted something—a favor, or an errand. I felt guilty and answered. The first thing that came was her breathing, then my name as if it were being dragged on glass. She was crying in the doctor's office and she needed me to pick her up. Months later I would call myself from her cell phone just to see that number flash once more.

I remember dressing, knocking over a glass, and I just left it. I found myself in the bathroom mirror, pulling my hair up. I pleaded with my reflection. I could fix this. I will stop at nothing when it comes to her.

The sound in her voice was one I had always feared though I had never heard it. It was the voice in a nightmare from my childhood when out of nowhere, in the soot of night, I understood that she would die.

I wrote canon that day in the bathroom. Made a religion with myself as god. A god was required to fix this, so I had to find one to believe in. I need a gate to fall down on tomorrow to buy me some time. But if I cannot save her, then she is not going to die alone. I saw her in my arms as the life crawled out and me telling her, *Count back from ten*, while she lets it out. And I have nothing better to say, nothing better to do than hold her as I lose her.

Run from the bathroom. Run down the long hall. And the house springs into position. The shoes again—I fall over them. The drawers, the closets are screaming. Run for the front door. Fall on the newspapers. Grab for the wall. The pictures come down. I shut the door and hear them smash. There is something on my mother's brain.

The cab pulled up to the doctor's office. The doors were heavy. In the corner of the waiting room were her huge eyes. She was slouching. She always did and told me to sit straight. She was reading the paper. She disliked being idle. I went and sat right in her lap.

When I was a child my mother would come home at night and lie down on the floor next to my bed. And in her charcoaled eyes and evening dress, her hands moving back and forth in the air above, my mother would tell me the story of the night.

We were two flies on the wall of the places she had been. We studied the strange conversations of adults, what they said and what they did not.

We were two shadows of performers on a stage. We whispered their lines along with them. Sometimes she would take me to a play she had described and I would watch the world follow my mother's words.

I have a memory or maybe just a dream. I watch her through the bars of my crib. Her black straight hair hangs down over one eye. Her two large hands she always hid. I chew on the wooden bars, leaving little teeth marks that are still there on the crib that's stored down in our basement. I was always trying to get closer to her.

As soon as I could coo, she started to solicit my advice. She confided in me, and maybe I responded every year with a more complete sentence. She expected that I would grow into the job. I had *a natural sensitivity*. I had *unusual intelligence*. I understood human interactions on my own little frequency, she said. She tapped messages and needed data back from me.

She found in me someone she had lost. Mother and child were intertwined in her and both of them were reborn in me. I often felt as a child that through me she was reaching back. Even very young I knew that I was being soothed for wounds not mine. My mother always said, *Each child is a visitor from another planet. You have to learn their customs.* But I think it was her customs that I learned.

She took me everywhere. I spent more time with adults than I did with children. She took me to lectures and interviews and meetings. She had a bag of toys for me to play with. *It's lucky for me*, she said, *I have a child who can dream anywhere she is.* I spent a large portion of my childhood underneath tables playing among the feet of strangers. My mother would lean down into my world, away from the other adults. I would grab her face. *You are mine, mine—mine.* We could talk secretly down there. I understood that even when she was momentarily pulled away, this woman belonged to me. She would pass down plates of food she had arranged like sculptures, smiley faces, a bird made of carrots. If I wanted more, I would tug on her dress.

When my mother was a child, she would tie her wrist to Irene's apron string when they took naps. This was to avoid ever being left behind. In some way she tied herself to me too. I was five when I said to her,

I just realized we are separate people.

What did you think? she asked.

That we were one person in two bodies.

She wrote this one down in her journal. *Worry?* Written in red sideways down the margin.

My mother could speak on any subject. It seemed she had read every book. Yet so much of her time was spent feeling worthless. As a child I thought that in private everyone was like this. I thought that being close meant helping someone dig themselves out of self-loathing. My mother would grow dark and still. Then it would pass and she would climb out, dropping the sadness like a rag. At times our closeness felt as if we had unraveled and become as weightless as ribbons. And each other's grip was the only thing that kept us from drifting away.

I was an anxious child. I rubbed my teddy's ears until they had no fur. When my mother left the house, I would remind her, *Don't stand too close to the curb. Look both ways. Call me from the pay phone.* I always felt that somehow I was keeping her alive.

The doctor came out of his office into the waiting room. He said we shouldn't assume it was a tumor on my mother's brain. He said it was the size of an almond. He had scheduled an MRI for her that afternoon.

We killed the hour before the MRI at an Italian restaurant on the Upper East Side, four blocks from the radiologist's office. I watched her try to enter through a window and exit through the bathroom. I quickly learned that I must always hold her hand. There are a million things that can hurt her—the corner of a table, a wall, a leaning umbrella. I watch people wonder what is wrong with her. At this point, she can still dress, and she is still beautiful. I think, what will they do if she gets ugly? Will she get ugly? I think how to protect her. We order and don't eat.

My father calls while we are at the table. I listen to her tell him not to come. He is traveling for work. We wouldn't know anything definitive until after he was supposed to come back anyway. She told him that he must stay calm. He never could sleep through the night. For years my mother would wake up to give him back rubs in the early hours of morning.

My three half sisters from my father's first marriage, Chris, Cindy, and Carole, were calling almost every hour. I imagined each of them with a packed bag by the door.

My mother had called my eldest sister, Chris, that very morning. My mother was starting to feel worried. She rattled off her symptoms to Chris (a nurse practitioner), who told her, *Run do not walk to the doctor.*

It was strange that my father kept dismissing my mother's symptoms as jet lag. Growing up I had severe headaches, and dozens of times we had ruled out spinal meningitis. I remember once I pretended to struggle to touch my chin to my chest so I could watch my dad freak out a little. But with my mother he must have had no room in his heart for this. She was his young wife, eleven years his junior. They had spent a great deal of time discussing her fear of losing him someday and his fear of leaving her behind.

My mother wanted to wait to call her little sister. She felt protective of Diane. They were extremely close, though at times their relationship was fraught. My mother always worried that she might lose Diane. In some ways she perceived Diane as she had Irene.

They let me sit in the room while she has her MRI. I touch her foot so she knows that I am there. The rest of her is hidden, pushed inside the yawning machine. It makes a sound like a hammer and drills.

They explain to her all that is going to happen. They point to the panic button, which I know she will never use. I know she will not open her eyes. She will travel elsewhere in her mind. I know she has already chosen where.

We are on a beach in late July. Perfect temperature. You, my fat healthy baby, are splashing in the surf, singing softly at my side in your broken English.

My mother is so still in that machine that I feel frightened. I tug her toe, as we had prearranged. She wiggles back. Most of my mother is not here. She traveled fast to another time. My mother is an athlete of the mind.

The next day I go to get the slides. I cross the park by bike, carrying the folder in my basket. I stop and pull the slides out to try to see something for myself. But the July sun blocks out all the black.

In the morning she woke up and cried for hours. She called my dad, and when she hung up, she said he was coming after all. My dad was home by midnight.

Cindy, Chris, Carole, and my mother were all worried over him. I found this annoying. I couldn't spare a thought for him. But they had reason to worry. At seventy-seven he was still working at a frenetic pace running his nonprofit. He traveled constantly, lecturing around the world. He enjoyed his work and equated retirement with death. However, he did plan on slowing down. He was looking for someone who could succeed him as CEO of his organization.

It was called the International Longevity Center. The focus of the center was promoting health in the growing aging population of America through policy, research, and education. The center was the culmination of his life's work as a physician, gerontologist, and writer. He had won a Pulitzer for his book published in 1975, *Why Survive? Being Old in America*. He was known around the world for his work on the social needs and rights of the elderly and his research on healthy aging and dementia. He had appeared before Congress, done hundreds of media interviews, both alone and with my mother at his side.

He had first recognized age discrimination as a young gerontologist and psychiatrist in 1968. He himself coined the term "ageism."

He had initiated the creation of the National Institute on Aging at the National Institutes of Health in Washington, D.C., and served as its first director. During his years there he and my mother cowrote their book *Love and Sex After Sixty*.

He moved us to New York in 1983 when I was three years old in order to establish the first department of geriatrics in a U.S. medical school, at Mount Sinai.

In 1995, President Bill Clinton named him chairman of the White House Conference on Aging.

My father was an exceptional man, a feminist who often chose to mentor women doctors. In fact his two main mentees became surrogate daughters numbers five and six. These women were young mothers whose child-care needs he understood and supported while he trained them.

Both these women would become successful doctors, and one of them would win a MacArthur "Genius Grant." They maintained a friendship with my father and my mother through the years.

His beloved personal assistant had a similar story. He started her workday at eleven so that she could spend the morning caring for her kids. His respect for the needs of working mothers was rooted in his memory of his grandmother, who raised him during the Depression. He often described her heroic struggle to keep them afloat after her husband's death.

And yet my father's feminism did not benefit the working mother with whom he lived. Maybe it would have cost him too much. His assumption that my mother would handle certain things was matched by her assumption that those things were hers to handle. In his personal life, he was very much a man of his generation. He left the family matters to her. She reminded him of children's birthdays and grandchildren's birthdays. She wrote all the cards and had him sign. She insisted on the college funds and special presents, the sensitive gifts and emotional interventions. It was she who nursed his aging mother, who managed the home and all my needs.

My mother was his greatest fan and his collaborator. She was devoted to him and his work. And yet behind this smiling pair there was a brooding woman, unfulfilled, unrecognized, kept from reaching her own apex in part by my father's dominant persona.

They wrote and lectured extensively together, but she always felt she was his sidekick. To some extent she wasn't wrong. She had joined the field of aging years after my father. Before meeting him her work had focused mainly on women. He influenced her and she idolized him. Dad had worked in that field before her. He was its major pioneer. Why did she expect to be considered at his level in the field in which he held so much expertise? She could conceivably have reached his level. She could have demanded more from him. The equality she craved she could have taken by force. He would have conceded. She was smart enough. She was hardworking enough. What she lacked was his confidence. She never felt she was enough.

There was no doubt in anyone's mind that she was his intellectual equal. Dad considered her the smartest, most exciting person he had ever met. She had everything it took to be his equal except the self-esteem.

Standing at his side did have its benefits. My mother was able to see life from his velocity. Yet while she enjoyed the world he opened up to her, she was threatened by his healthy sense of self that powered him along.

This lack meant that my father overruled her. His agenda always won. Whether it was her tome on women's history that he had promised to co-write with her and never did or the evidence in our closet of her contribution to his Pulitzer, a copy of the manuscript for *Why Survive?* covered in her writing. My father was a man you had to match. He was self-centered. He lived in a sort of fever, a scrambling to work, dreaming of work. His days were spent in a state of flow, lifted by his passion with no time to worry over the dreams of the woman beside him. Like many natural leaders, he knew how to delegate, and like many men—especially of his generation—he sometimes mistook his wife's work for his own.

My mother played her part, keen to hide in my father's shadow, afraid of the limelight for the scrutiny it held. My father gave her access to a rarified world, and she let herself believe that he was the reason she belonged there. My mother was extremely competitive, a hardworking person. It was what had delivered her so far from where she had begun. But when she met my father, she mistook a colleague for a mentor. She never did let go of that perception.

As generous as she was and as focused on the needs of other people, my mother longed for the same level of recognition that my father received. In some ways my father was her victim, an externalized enemy that she did not recognize was coming from within. In other ways she was my father's victim. He had few insecurities and this amazing focus. He had work that he loved, work that was altruistic, generative, fulfilling.

She had been braver and stronger in her youth. The solitude that she had felt in childhood was part of what drove her to excel in school, in sports, and eventually at college. Yet by the time I came along, it seemed that her ambition had become eclipsed by doubt, insecurity, and guilt, and what was once a drive to succeed in her own life had become a competition with my dad. There was never a time that I remember when she wasn't angry with him or with herself in relationship to him. She blamed him for making her feel bad about herself, and with my child's judgment, I blamed my father too. My father was not innocent. Like so many successful men, he knew how to delegate. My mother was the opposite. She had a funny habit of doing other people's work for them and giving them all the credit for it.

When I was in fifth grade, she won me a science prize for a project on the ozone layer. My parents were on sabbatical during that time, writing a book, and we were living in Switzerland for eleven months. I felt so ashamed as I crossed the auditorium of the girl's boarding school where I was a day student. I felt like everybody knew. I wonder now if my father ever felt this way.

Had he been a different man, less self-centered, he might have cared more for her in the right way, and yet in so many ways she was impossible. She was inconsolable. She had decided. It was her choice to live his way. For his attentiveness, his investment in her work would never match the level of her interest in his. In that way, both my parents fell short of their vision for the world.

July thirteenth. The slides lay on the doctor's desk. We sat waiting in his office. Chris had come up from D.C. She and Dad were clutching my mother's hands. There was dread on our faces as we smiled at one another in the small, choked office on the high floor. My mother kept asking me if I was okay. She kept wrapping her arms around me tighter and tighter, and the cell phone was ringing in my bag, then in her bag, then in my father's and sister's. And the room was animated by fear.

The doctor came and asked some long and detailed questions, and then I saw my first neurological exam. She was to touch her nose with one hand, then the other, walk in a line, and several other things. It seemed that she was passing, and for a moment the expression on my father's face was hopeful, and I could feel myself inching forward through the taut air in the room to see her clearly.

The doctor said, *You may sit down.* He said it was clear to him what this was, but he could not be completely certain until it was taken out. He said the worst-case scenario was . . . a *glioblastoma,* Chris finished his sentence.

I looked it up online. *Glioblastoma multiforme (GBM) is the most common, deadliest malignant primary brain tumor. It is a grade IV astrocytoma with star-shaped glial cells called astrocytes that infiltrate the surrounding brain tissue. Complete surgical removal is not possible. The cause is unknown though research points increasingly to genetic mutations.*

The doctor shows us scans. It is on her right occipital lobe, which I learn is the lower back portion of the brain. He tells us pressure produced by the growth is in itself life threatening irrespective of the nature of the growth. In other words, whatever this is, it must be taken out immediately. He says that if he can find a surgeon, the procedure will be done in the next twenty-four hours. Brain surgery. Two days before her sixty-fifth birthday.

I remember wondering what would happen if we just left the thing in—whether her brain would explode and run out her eyes. I was so ignorant and it was so macabre, so science fiction, as normal life walked out on us that day.

Doctor, I need you to tell me what I should do with my baby.

I was ashamed when she said it. Ashamed when she cried it out. I felt overgrown in my seat, and yet like a terrified child clinging to my mother's skirt. *She is going to die,* I thought. I knew.

The doctor said the growth was bigger than an almond. More like a walnut with its shell. He said that she showed signs of serious brain damage. She started to ramble then, as if trying to string together thoughts as proof that she was sane. As if trying to show that whatever we are made of—the soul, the mind was still working, still standing straight and strong, stamping its feet against the ground of herself, calling out, *Solid earth here!*

He told her she had lost the vision on the left side of both her eyes. This is what her eye exam revealed. And then I noticed the sheets of white paper with her name and the name of her eye doctor—devious messengers lying hidden among the clutter on his desk. He explained that her loss of vision was due to the growth pressing down on her ocular nerve. She piped up that she had known this but that her eye doctor had told her that she would regain it. The neurologist just shook his head.

I found myself looking around the room for these people I still thought of as *adults* to set things right. All were still. All were crying. I couldn't recall if I had ever seen my father cry. He moved to say something. I held my breath, waiting for the words that would carry this away. But all he said was, *Can I take her home?*

I looked down at her hands. And tried to memorize them. My father straightened up. He asked Chris if she had been taking notes. He started to speak like a doctor with the neurologist. They plotted out the next few days. There was talk of treatment and of timing. But I could not make sense of the words.

We took the elevator down. My mother and father held hands side by side, their backs pressed up against the wall as we plunged down. They stared straight ahead, moons for eyes, a bride and groom. I jumped then, fell all the way onto the street. I chose my grief over their agony, over their hope.

We hailed a cab for home, so that she could collect her things for the hospital. It was storming. I called my aunt Diane from the apartment. I told her there was something on my mother's brain but that we didn't know what it was yet. I heard the phone drop and the sound of her voice screaming her husband's name.

My mother was wrapping little shampoo bottles in plastic like she always did, taking time to twist red wires around the tops. She packed some of her work papers, books that she was reading.

The storm was shaking the apartment. Things were flying against the window—city things, like plastic bags. She had always loved storms, but now nothing felt real. I had nothing to do while my mother packed, so I kept calling different people to tell them what had happened. This made me feel better. I was soothed to hear them upset. I felt I was starting to go numb, drifting into another state not quite of the living. I needed to feel the reaction of the living.

There was a storm when I was little, in my mother's hometown in Minnesota. I was at my cousin Athena's. We stood at the edge of her family's cornfield, looking out over the wind and weather. She was braiding my hair. I had my grandpa's shirt on and was stuffed into borrowed Keds with missing laces. I had left my sneakers at the bottom of the creek. I was ten.

A tornado was headed our way. My mother and grandfather were coming for me. I could see the old Buick moving on the other side of the cornfield, racing down the long, thin road, throwing up clouds of dust. Grandpa was driving fast—racing the tornado. They should have left me at Athena's, but my mother wanted me with her.

All the animals were going mad and making sounds. The dogs were running short sprints back and forth between the house and the barn. Grandpa's car turned the corner to come toward us, then he disappeared a few seconds just beyond a hill, but I could see the dust rising and I knew how close he was. They pulled the car right up and pulled me in without stopping. Athena's mother picked her up and ran into their house. We raced back. I held my head out the window as we flew home, the wind unraveling the carefully twisted braid.

The surgeon couldn't perform the operation until the following Monday, and she had to stay in the hospital until then. Thursday passed with the arrival of my two other sisters, Carole and Cindy, various tests, and blood work.

As usual, Carole was in some fancy hotel on Central Park South. She always made sure to keep a distance, never staying with us. She adored our father and yet seemed satisfied to see him once a year.

She and her mother had always been at odds. My mom had tried to nurture Carole, but none of us could get her to stay still or submit. She was always asserting that distance. Yet today she sat at the edge of the hospital bed with no sign of leaving.

Chris and Cindy were, as usual, at our house. Like Chris, Cindy had brought a notebook to record everything the doctors said. Chris (*the brilliant nurse practitioner*, my mother announced to every doctor, nurse, nurse's aide who came into the room) stood at attention. She would assure my mother periodically that everything was being handled in the correct way.

My mother's veins were thin and hard to prick, and so her arms turned black and blue with the concentrated stabs of nurses.

I can tell just by looking at you that you are going to be good at this, she said to each one before they butchered her arm. She believed that through positive reinforcement she would receive better treatment. This was partly true. Of course, kindness cannot make up for lack of skill on the part of another, but it did mean that almost every person who entered that room arrived with affection for my mother.

Everyone was greeted with a smile, as if she had been waiting for their particular arrival. On a third or fourth visit, an individual would be greeted with a hug and joyous hello. She was quickly well versed on the personal lives of several of her visiting doctors and residents.

She had a sincere interest in everyone with whom she came into contact. She never forgot details. She memorized you. This had been what drew her to the field of social work—a voracious lifelong study of people.

We've got to find you a woman, she would say to one.

It's the hours I work, he would reply. *Women can't take it.*

But you, she would counter, *are so gentle, and look at this bed. You know how to make hospital corners. Just give me some time to think it over. A man who knows how to make hospital corners is the next model of man.*

She volunteered as show-and-tell for a class of neurology students. I hated the idea, but I wasn't surprised. Goddamn if she wasn't going to spend her day putting a *human face on cancer*. Now she could feel like a professional in place of a patient.

I accompanied her grumpily, along with Carole and Chris. My mother saluted the students upon entry, and I followed just behind her, scrutinizing their faces. I wanted to kill them—all those smug, young people. They didn't even know who my mother was. One of them yawned as he opened his notebook.

Typical Friday, I guess, you son of a bitch.

My mother was given what now felt like her twentieth neurological exam, since every resident and doctor that had entered her hospital room over the past twenty-four hours had asked her to touch her nose or walk in a straight line heel to toe.

Put your hand over your eye, the professor said. *How many fingers am I holding up?* My mother got the answer wrong, and the professor spun around on his heels. *Yes!* he exclaimed with great zeal. *Now what does this tell us?* The class laughed at the passion of their spirited teacher, and a mob of hands shot up. *Just a typical Friday's class, I guess.*

I remember the words, scientific explanations, most of which I didn't understand. I remember a young, French doctor passing me a note that was rather flirtatious. I remember my sister Carole at the front of the room.

Carole could have been a neurologist, my mother began saying that day. Carole had never, to my knowledge, considered the medical profession. Furthermore, she seemed quite happy without a career. But my mother was not happy. She felt Carole was too smart and my mother kept a mental Rolodex of people's unlived lives.

I saw my mother smile at Carole from her chair in front of the note board. I remember the back of Carole's head. Her blond hair was tied up, her back arched forward over the desk. She did look quite engaged.

I looked at my sister Chris. She was watching my mother. Like me, she had been crying for days. Her face was locked in hope and desperation contained behind a smile she kept directing at my mother—a nod of the head, a look of knowing pride when my mother would answer a question in a humorous way, making the class giggle. Looking at my sisters, I felt I saw them for the first time, through my mother's eyes.

I recall only a happy family, but this had not always been the case. My mother had joined the family at a complicated time. My father's marriage to his first wife was unhappy. My parents always refused to tell me how they met. And this has always made me uncertain that I want to know.

My mother had been married once before, but she divorced. She married my father in 1972 and I was born eight years later. It took her a while to convince him to have another child. He said she told him she wanted two things, one was a Ph.D., the other was a baby. She promised she would take care of me mostly on her own—a strange, redundant promise for a woman of her generation to make.

I have heard whispers about timing. When my father's marriage ended in relation to when he started his story with Mom. The details alter depending on whose telling it is. The story that I choose is the one my mother told.

She was a social worker in a hospital in Washington, D.C. A young woman walked into the psych ER one day, surrounded by her children. She pleaded for admittance, but the doctor on call did not believe her, and she was turned away. She walked down to the highway, leaving her small children at the edge, holding hands like dolls in the tall grass. She walked into the traffic.

The hospital was sued over her death, and my father, as a member of the board, was consulted on the case. The assumption was that he would back the hospital, but he took the other side and in the process, he won my mother's heart. This story is who my parents are. Even if it's not completely true. Even if they were already seeing one another, this is how my parents would have met.

At first my sisters hated my mother and were furious with Dad. Chris threatened to forget the family altogether. Carole had already begun to withdraw. Cindy was the first one to come around. After college, she moved home to complete a yearlong internship. During that year, she and my mother slowly became friends.

It is strange, considering my mother's entrance as the other woman, but my mother started helping my dad repair the damage with his girls. She convinced him to have weekly dinners alone with Chris. At first they went to restaurants, but Chris grew tired of crying in public, so my mother would have a dinner prepared, light candles in the dining room, set two places at the table, and shut the double doors. Chris and Dad would be in there for hours, the hum of their voices occasionally spiking in crescendo.

My mother always saw people as children. As if they were Russian dolls, she would peel them down to their smallest form and meet them there with outstretched arms. Her developing friendship with each of my sisters was informed by her reading of their needs and tailored to each individually. My mother was not a one-size-fits-all lady; instead she shape-shifted to connect. Sometimes she contorted into unhealthy positions, as with her own sister.

With my sisters she held their mother firmly in her mind. Each of them had had a vastly different experience as a daughter. My mother understood this. It was the same with her and her siblings.

By the time I was born everyone could smile down at me. I was passed around. I never felt as if I were the fruit of two home wreckers. I was be-loved, surrounded by people who loved each other. My sisters began to have their babies; six nieces and nephews became like my brothers and sisters, my best friends.

My mother always told me to stay close to my sisters. She was older, she said, and would not be here forever. *Never grow apart*, she said.

The professor asked my mother to walk a line from the note board to the back of the classroom. The students were having their lunch during the class. There was a buffet by the side window. They took great bites and chewed either thoughtfully or absentmindedly as they watched my mother pass. She was concentrating on a spot she had picked on the back wall, a focal point. Unlike all these students with all their knowledge, I knew her. I knew what she saw on that back wall. She was struggling, walking toward her life. I saw her body shake every time she moved one foot forward. She bit her lip as she matched up toe to heel. Her hands were spread, the fin-gers strained against their webbing, her skeleton moved forward in space, searching desperately for balance, finding strength in memory, drawing from every step she'd taken in her life. She was sweating and breathing and taking a step, sweating and breathing and taking one more. And the students sat and ate and watched and whispered to each other.

When the class was over, I wanted to scream. I wanted to take a scythe and run it from one wall to the other, picking up heads like peas on a knife. But my mother just bowed.

I wish you all great success! she cried as my sisters took her hands and led her from the room.

There is no word, like "gentleman," to describe a lady. "Gentlewoman" doesn't ring the same. If a woman could be dapper, my mother was a Fred Astaire.

Friday came and with it her sixty-fifth birthday. My father asked her doctors if we could take her out for a while. She wanted to go to the park. She was in love with Central Park.

When I was little she would walk me through the park, pointing out all the species of bird, animal, of tree and flower, picking up earth between her fingers. After her father died, she would go to Central Park to think of him. She would come back hours later and tell us what the park was doing—as if it were gossip that flowers were blooming or some tree had been chopped down. She kept track of the ducklings in the pond and noted their development, or lack of maturation—how one seemed to lag behind the others.

There would come a time when I would take to standing by her window. I would look out onto the park and imagine I could see her moving down there, that I could see her through the trees, that she was only hiding from me.

On her sixty-sixth birthday we took pictures in which all of us are crying. My three sisters, my father, and I, and my niece curled up in my mother's arms. We found ourselves at the Conservatory Garden. They had started her on steroids, and she was sweating in the sun. She hung on her bones like a rag. She seemed to be chasing old memories from garden to garden. And each one was her favorite.

We took great swigs from a bottle of water that we passed between hands as we went in various groups of twos and threes led by my mother, her head cocked forward, all eyes and nose, all seeing and smiling and drinking in every flower of each garden, storing life up. The tips of her fingers rubbed together, like her whole body was savoring air and sun and every footstep that she took; every footstep around her rang in her ears. *I can hear everything*, she said.

She had told my sister Cindy that she could handle whatever this was. On the phone when she had called to say that there was something on her brain, she said, *I think I can handle this.* But when my sister had arrived, my mother said, *Please forget what I told you.* And Cindy held her in the folds of gray hospital, in the discouraging smell of the food, in the rush of white coats and eager residents, the sterile smell of birth and death, the factory of life, the input and output of humans in which my mother was at present lost. None of us knew which way she was going. We knew only that this was too close for comfort, to the edge of the unknown. This was too much out of our hands and out of the hands of a person who had always cared for us.

In the Conservatory Garden, we were dazed in the heat. Most of us had slept in the hospital. Some of us had bathed. My mother's loss of vision, the new drugs, and the heat combined to make her unsteady on her feet. That day I put my arm out many times to catch her as she fell.

There was a wedding party being photographed in one of the gardens. My mother stopped to watch and clasped her hands. *Oh look how exciting this is!* She stepped into the frame, halting the wedding picture. The people didn't seem to mind. They were all primping and talking as she moved among them wearing her wide smile. I could see that she wasn't herself. She seemed stoned, in a state of free association.

She began to flirt with the young couple. They were all very good-natured at first. For a few minutes they thought she was sweet, but then I saw that they thought she was strange, and in my head I damned their marriage. I killed their children, then reconsidered and gave them an illness. Let it be drawn-out pain. I wished for them to see my mother's image when they wondered why such bad luck had befallen their family. I cursed them with all the abandon of silence.

This is wonderful, my mother was saying. *What an exciting time this is!* And she realized that she was blocking the picture, and she put out her hand as if to apologize, but the bride took it, and the two women stood face-to-face. There was no noise: the only conversation was the meeting of their eyes.

I wish you great joy, my mother said and turned to go, and the wedding party slowly resumed.

The cab was racing through the park to the East Side. He wasn't a good driver—the turns and curves were too sharp. You kept bouncing around, and you were crying.

I said, *We don't know what this is yet.*

I was being controlling. I was gripping your arm.

It's stupid to cry. We don't know what this is.

I am yelling.

This could be a cyst. This could be a cyst.

Reprimanding.

Don't do this to yourself. Don't do this to me.

Pain has a boiling point at which it will turn into anger or silence.

We had gotten permission to take you from the hospital even though you were having brain surgery in two days. It was your birthday. The last thing we did that day was go to the movies because you were getting hot in the sunlight. You were overheating, you were pumped full of steroids—your first day.

At the movies my niece spilled hot nacho cheese all down your front, and I wanted to beat her face in. I cleaned you in the bathroom. You were crying in the stall like a pig on your brother's farm. The world was a slaughterhouse. I could see you through the slim gap of the metal door. Without laying down toilet paper, you sat right down. You said it wasn't worth it, and I threw up in the sink.

The words of the living are useless. The living can't help but be blind, distracted by the objects of life—the people, the pavement and trees, the plans and the future, the water and food and babies, neon lights, and comfort.

When you were leaving the bathroom, a woman was coming in, and you walked into her. I was behind you, trying to guide you, but in your panic you were rushing, and she balked. She must have realized after that you were not well, and she followed us outside to apologize. You were sobbing when my father led you out, and I turned to her and pointed at her pregnant belly.

Good luck with that, I said.

Mom's surgery was to take place on the fifteenth floor of the hospital, but for some reason I remember it taking place in the basement. For some reason, I thought we left her in the basement that day, in the cellar. *The cellar*, I remember thinking. The words ran laps around my mind. *The cellar*. The morning of her surgery, I woke up and threw up.

They had wrapped her head the night before in white gauze right over her hair. She looked like a ghastly vision of a bride. It made no sense. Apparently they didn't need to shave her head completely. They would just cut and pull the scalp back—hair and all. And *hair and all* joined the *cellar* in running laps.

The night before her surgery was rough. She was stoned. She was swearing and itching and writhing in her bed. She spoke in her sleep about violent things, about killing and *you shut up* and *you can go to hell*. I trembled in the corner on my cot, a little girl. *She doesn't mean it* repeating in my head. My sister Chris slept upright in a chair. Every so often she would whisper soothing words. My mother told Chris that she could go and fuck herself, and in my pulse pounded the words *this is not my mother*.

The next morning, it seemed that she remembered nothing of the night before. We took turns climbing into bed with her. It felt Catholic, like we were climbing into the confessional. There was whispering between my mother and us all. It was like a benediction, as if she were blessing us, each and every one while we paid our last respects. She would hold your face in her hands and tell you how sorry she was. I remember my sister Cindy sitting on my mother's bed. Her hair was coming out of her ponytail. She was hunched over my mother, and she looked twenty years younger than she really was. Cindy had lost a little brother when she was only four.

He was my father's only son, the son of his first wife. He died after two weeks in the hospital, never coming home, and my father, in his pain, folded into himself. The four-year-old did not receive enough explanation or understand the meaning of all that had happened, and the strain of the experience remained, a legacy of childhood. My mother knew this, had pointed it out to my father, and made him address it with the four-year-old who was now an adult.

As Cindy sat crying on her bed, I remember my mother saying, *Now I can help you get over your fear of death.* Her bravado enraged me. My mother always thought that she had superpowers when it came to healing other people. And it was true that she was gifted, but what she really ended up with were legions of adopted children, because people want love above all else. And above all else, my mother longed to give it.

They came for her around noon to take her down to the basement, where the surgical staff was already preparing. My father and I clutched the sides of the gurney, holding her strong, warm hands. The attendants pushing the gurney looked overworked and underpaid and grumpy as they pulled and pushed her along. The gurney kept getting banged against the doorframes, and she kept repeating, *It's okay. It's okay.*

The anesthesiologist thought herself hilarious. We tried to laugh as if to stay in her good graces. We were leaving a treasure in her care. My dad kept turning his head away to cry. I guess he didn't want to scare my mother, but I cried outright, even when the surgical team glared and shook their heads. I cried as hard as I could. No one here was stupid. We all knew what was at stake. And then when she was still awake, still whispering kind words to us, we had to leave her there, alone.

The tumor was on the right occipital lobe of her brain. The procedure was called a craniotomy. We were told that the risk of stroke, paralysis, infection, hemorrhage, blood clot, and pneumonia was low but nevertheless real. I can't recall how long it lasted—maybe six, maybe seven hours.

I went home and lay in my parents' bed, the closest I could get. I now understood true helplessness not perceived, not invented. And all at once out of my despair rose a strange euphoria, a freedom from family, identity, from self. I had a sense of what I was before my birth—some anterior state. I hovered there a moment, looking down over my life and my own suffering without any emotion.

My body lay in my mother's bed as the neurosurgeon made his first incision, pulling the skin and muscle off her bone and folding them back. He drilled holes in her skull, sawed off a section called the bone flap, and lifted that new separate piece off from her head. He sliced through the dura mater—a thin membrane that protects the brain—placed retractors around the opening, and began his work on the resection of the tumor.

When the procedure was complete, the retractors removed, the dura mater sutured, the bone flap secured, and the muscles and skin sewn back, they placed a white gauze turban once again over my mother's head. And then she came drifting—drifting in her white sheet past the white walls back toward my body.

My mother had a dry sense of humor. She used it to gain a measure of control over my dad. He could be the star out in the world, but he was not allowed to be in our family of three. She made fun of him. She put him down. She would charm him into submission. She could make him curl up at her feet like a lion turned house cat. Then she would pass my dad to me. Whether he required this kind of wrangling has only recently become a question in my mind. On some level she was ever waging war on him, and I seemed to be the object of dispute.

I never got the chance to know my father for myself. I met him through the eyes of the other women in his life. Between my mother and sisters there were so many stories. His crimes were tsk-tsked about for years. I wonder how I would have looked upon him had I ever been able to judge him for myself. My concept of my father, up through my early twenties, was cloaked in the thick folds of my mother's mythology.

There was the famous story of the ice cream scoop. My mother gave Cindy an ice cream scoop that she and my father never used. When my dad found out, he lost his mind. How dare they give away his ice cream scoop! There was shouting on both sides. The argument harked back to several years before when he had refused to loan Cindy a couple hundred bucks that would allow her to go to Africa. She had been working several jobs and saving for two years.

Then there was Chris's story about how Dad took her to a cocktail party and then left her standing alone by the bar.

Allegedly he once refused to give Cindy money for the movies because he said that if he did he would not be able to afford to go himself. Cindy was thirteen at the time. My mother never contextualized my father's behavior. He was in the midst of divorce, completely broke, and up to his neck in debt, his first wife taking her revenge with his credit card.

Yes, my dad was funny about money, probably due in part to his Depression childhood. He could act like the cheapest man in the entire world. Yes, he was driven and self-centered. He had a temper. But so did his daughters.

I know it is easy to romanticize the one that got away. Yet for me the placing of my father on a pedestal is a new and radical act. When I was five, I asked him if he would marry me because I'd heard somewhere that's what daughters always do. I recall the feeling of lying to my father's face about how much I loved him. My mother always told me not expect too much from him. She told me to love him for what he was and get from her all the things he wasn't. Wonderful as my mother was in many ways, too much was exactly what she gave me.

My mother did want my father and me to be close, but she felt our closeness depended on her. She had to move us away from our natural state, which in her mind was one of discord and alienation. I don't know where she got this idea. I don't know what was true and what was false. I know she believed she was doing the right thing for us both.

So I was never a daddy's girl. Being mommy's girl was too demanding. He and I always had a natural and special connection, yet in my heart I always held him at a distance.

I woke up tangled in the sheets. There was no message on my phone. I thought of how she had found ways to thank me, all my life, for being born. She had always expressed this gratitude at the chance to have a child. She had waited forty-two years, and I, through luck of birth, grew up always in her joy and welcome. I thought of this and cried until I slept again, cell phone in my hand, waiting to be summoned back to the hospital and to her side.

The ring. The cab. The curb. The rotating door. The family in the waiting room. My father was seated, rigidly, trying to read his work papers. My father was incapable of inactivity. His life was characterized by hyper-productivity, especially during difficult times.

He credited his passion for his work to the sudden death of his grandfather when he was only seven. This man was the closest thing to a dad my father ever had. He never knew his father, who abandoned him when he was young. His mother, Easter, was working as a showgirl in New York City. Before she had brought him to her mother's house the two of them had been homeless for a short time. They spent their final night together sleeping in Grand Central Station. Then she brought him to her parents and was gone.

My father remembered following his grandfather around, going with him to the back yard, where they fed their chickens. When his grandfather died, they told my father that he had merely gone away. My father was silent many days, thinking deeply, until it slowly dawned on him that his grandfather had died. In that moment, he decided that had he been a doctor, he could have saved his grandfather. So he became one.

He was so well connected in the medical field that I think they both believed whatever she ended up having he could save her. And he tried. As with everything, he threw himself into the task of keeping my mother alive.

The kind of devastating loss that had informed his life lay before him again. In a matter of days he grew older. His face changed. It was suddenly, drastically distorted in the waiting room as we were paged to the office of the neurosurgeon.

The neurosurgeon was on the phone as we ran into his office. My sisters, my father, and I sat all around the room. We didn't think to drag the chairs to close formation, and after we sat, we kept inching toward one another as the surgeon finished his conversation. Finally, the phone hit the cradle, and he raised his face to us.

Cancer. Tumor. Glioblastoma. Stage four. No cure. His and our job was to make her death as painless as possible. She had six to eighteen months.

The tentacles of the tumor crawl from its nucleus through my mother's brain. The tentacles or fingers are miniscule, microscopic. You can't find them with the naked eye. After pulling the tumor from her brain and holding it under magnification, he could see where it was ripped from its fingers. They were still running through her brain, sly messengers hidden within.

They erased the days and rolled them out behind me; my mother was a person from my past, a gift that I had taken for granted. She would never know my child, never meet my partner, never let her hair grow white, never grow old by a fire and drift off into what only felt like sleep.

He gave us the library next to his office to recover while we waited to see her. The room was consumed by a wood table; a heavy slab that cut right through its center.

My sisters wavered, waiting to see where our father would sit. They were staring at him as if at any minute he would fall. He sat. I sat across from him. He was folded inward. He kept repeating, *I can save her*. This man slumped in the chair—I didn't know him. He was like another child, frightened and helpless.

My sisters put their arms around him. I wanted to scream at them, *This is happening to me too!* I felt I didn't love him as they did. I was so angry at him for not even turning to face me. Not even extending his hand. Did he feel he owed me nothing as a father? Would it be about only his pain? When he did not reach for me, some essential part of me flew off. I was sitting in for a self that was no longer whole.

A glioblastoma is a tremendous occurrence. It is a blue whale. It is a flood, submerging continents. If a brain were like the earth's surface, a glio would be a billion years of ecological change. And I watched a billion years come down on her. Through the falling debris I saw the flash of my mother's eyes disappear down a dark well into death's indefinable promise. There was a wave that washed over our family that would take her in its wake, screaming and scratching for the land. And all our love for her could do was watch.

They moved her from the operating room to the intensive care unit. I thought of how to tell her she would die. People kept telling me that it was not my job to tell her. I had no response. There was no one else. My father was not ready. Of this I was certain. And for some reason I did not understand, I found I was.

I went into the ICU to see her with my father. She was barely awake. We were amazed that she was awake at all. My father and I bent over her from opposite sides of the bed and put our faces to her neck. She was mumbling, active under the sheets. Her fingers were crawling, searching for us. Her face was propped up. It was almost levitating over the pillow. And when she heard my voice, her fingers came, padding and pulling on the sheets searching for me. When her hands found me, she pulled me to her and looped her arm around my head, threw the limp arm over me with all the force of her back, and drew me down. The mumbling got louder as she pulled me toward her, unable to open her eyes, unwilling to let go. *Say something,* I said. *Are you okay?* She kept cooing. I knew that she was worried about me. I kept asking, *Can you hear me? Can you hear me?* She said, *Headache.*

I spent the night with her in the ICU. I tried to lie with her, but the wires and plugs left me no room on the narrow bed. I dragged in a chair, but the nurse kicked me out to the waiting room—something about safety rules. I set my watch for every two hours until morning in order to check on her. It was a long night, hellish to sleep, hellish to wake. I would push through the heavy door into the ICU, unable to see a thing through my contacts, now shriveled dry against my eyes. The hospital air was cold and dense. It poured through the grates and dragged its icy fingers over us. It felt like we were captives on a ghost ship, now sealed and sunken on the ocean floor.

He was just here . . . she'd be talking when I came in. I could barely pull sentences from the ruin of words and grunts she made. Her fingers were like ice. I pulled another rough, thin sheet from the rolling shelves that had been parked by her bed. It angered me to deal with this. She was covered in three thin sheets replete with one anemic blanket that was really a sheet in disguise. She spoke again . . . *he hurt me.*

I scanned the hallway of the ICU for men, doctors, cleaning staff, but I saw no one. I was frightened to leave her. I tried pushing a chair far back against the wall to hide myself behind the curtain, but slowly, icily, came the nurse's hand to my shoulder, through the curtain. *I'm not going to tell you again. If I tell the head nurse, you will get kicked out of here.*

It was so late, and there were so many of them—eight or nine all along the ward. Some of them writhed in their beds. One of them kept calling out for someone. I wanted to carry my mother out of there. I wanted to carry her over the years to a time when all her family was around her, and she was strong and well and standing in the center, bathed in golden light, warm from food and heat, with eyes wide open.

I bent over her. She hadn't opened her eyes since the surgery. Her mouth kept whispering words of stress, reports of pain and abuse. When I touched her hand, she took mine fast, and I didn't want to take it back, to leave her, to drag myself back to the waiting room.

The next time I woke up, night had left, the sky was purple, and the night nurse had been replaced by a more kind one who was rather focused on her breakfast. I seized the chance and made my way into my mother's room, taking my seat against the wall and taking her hand.

Time passed, and it was morning rounds. I used my position at the wall to spy on doctors as they passed my mother, making their comments. I realize that in the quiet of an empty hallway, doctors admit to each other the mistakes they have made. Doctors always flex their rushed terminology at me, refuse to give me time, and when they give me time it just feels wasted.

My father arrived, taking my mother's hand where I left it for him on the bed.

After a day, she was moved from the intensive care unit to the neurological ward. My sisters said good-bye. They had been away from home and work for a while and had to return. They assured her they would be back. Cindy was the last to hug her, and then I saw Cindy turn before she burst into tears and hurried down the hallway.

I spent a night with her there, and the following day the doctors were already discussing sending her home. As it turns out, these days brain surgery warrants only a twenty-four-hour stay.

In the end they decided to keep her in the hospital another night. They wanted to be *overly cautious*. Despite the shrieking of the nurses, I stayed again, on a cot I brought from home. She had a roommate—a Haitian woman with bone cancer. She spoke no English, and no one spoke Creole. When she was agitated, they found a French-speaking doctor to explain things to her and inquire as to what she needed.

My dad tells me that bone cancer is one of the most painful types of cancer. I watch this woman. She is quiet. Her TV is never on. She lies and stares ahead except when her niece arrives bringing her flowers.

I walk my mother to the bathroom several times a day and night. We wave to the woman. We whisper how bad we feel for her—as if we were in such a good state ourselves. She nods her head when she sees me walking my mother around. The three of us speak like we understand each other's words. My mother always tries to give her chocolate, and she likes that. We always say good night before drawing the curtain between us. She blows us a kiss.

It was 4:00 A.M. when I walked my mother to the bathroom. She still had the white bandage around her head from after surgery. I hated to think of what was under it—a thread that kept the skin of my mother's scalp from rolling back.

I held her up in the bathroom and washed her hands and wrists. I tucked her back in bed and put the rumbling things around her legs. The rumbling things were plastic tubes that wrapped around the legs and trembled to stimulate the circulation and protect against clotting. I think of how Grandma Irene died of a blood clot after knee surgery—at least that's what we think happened. Shortly after coming home, she collapsed into my grandfather's arms and died.

I fall asleep. I can never get comfortable on hospital sheets rough as sandpaper. It is almost morning. Soon my dad will come. I'm in and out of consciousness. Maybe an hour goes by.

Maybe it is 5:00 A.M. when the strange noise starts. I keep my eyes closed. It is a wet noise like a finger in a wound. I see she has pulled the bandage off. She stirs the gaping hole, her finger in her head. I try to run into the hall, but my legs won't move. I start to struggle with her, but I cannot pull her finger from the hole. She is pulling out bits of her brain.

I wake up. I am struggling with sheets. I sit up at 5:15 A.M. She has her back to me. She is lying in bed. I call her name. She is very still, and then the noise again. I crawl up onto the bed toward her. I turn her toward me. She only sees ceiling. Her eyes are fixed. I call to her. The left side of her mouth is moving. It has become a separate entity, while the rest of her face stays still.

Suddenly, she asks me why I'm screaming. I want her to look at me. I tell her this. She moves her eyes slowly and holds my hand. She says, *I'm sorry, baby. I'll make it better.*

The nurse comes in and looks frightened. I ask her to help. She leaves. Another comes in, asks how long she has been like this. She leaves to call the doctors. She looked terrified. My mother asks what is happening. I tell her that her mouth is moving in a strange way. I tell her not to worry. I won't let anything happen to her. I think she is going to die.

The first nurse comes and looks without approaching the bed. I am screaming at her. *Do something!*

She turns to leave. I am begging her to stay. I think I will vomit. The Haitian woman is speaking in Creole, has opened the curtain, is reaching out—is crying. I pick up the phone, I drop it—my hands are shaking. I find it again, blindly fumbling with my fingers.

I am dialing Dad's number and holding my mother's hand. Her mouth stops for a while, and then starts again, stronger. She says she feels strange—like she can't control her mouth. She is trying to reach for it with her hand, but she can't find her face. There is blood on her teeth. I am dialing, but he won't pick up. I am going to be sick.

The nurse comes back in. She walks slowly toward the bed as if she would catch the plague, as if the bed were spitting flames. She says the resident has been called and is on his way. I motion to her. I reach out. I crack the phone on the table. *Help us!* I cover my mouth with my hand. I am screaming. I will scare my mother. I turn my back to my mother.

More of her is moving. Her shoulder is jerking up and down. Her mouth—her eyes are fixed.

What is happening to me?

Mommy! Mommy!

I'm sorry, Alex. I can't stop my mouth . . . mouth . . . mouth . . . mouth . . . mouth . . .

I am falling off the bed. I land on my stomach, swallow my vomit, and pull myself back up. Her eyes begin to roll back. I lay across her. I am shaking up and down with her.

Help us!

She grows still. I have been dialing home with my other hand. My father answers the phone. He is half asleep. He is coming. He doesn't know how serious this is. He worries that he won't find a cab. I am screaming to him on the phone. He doesn't get it. He is mad at me. She starts again: more of her this time, the whole left side of her body. She is saying his name, over and over again. He can hear her. I hear his phone hit the table and the sound of him running. I put the phone back in its cradle. She must be dying, so I put my face to her face.

She tries to whisper to me. Words of comfort run with blood. Words come out in hopeful eyes, pleading eyes.

Everything you do is perfect, Mom. You could never hurt me. I'm okay. We'll be all right. I wonder should I smother her.

She is no longer able to speak. I tell her she is the most precious thing to me. Nothing she could ever do would hurt me. The blood is on the bed now. The Haitian woman can't stand up, but she is trying. I think something has gone wrong with the surgery. I am losing my vision. I see the window at the end of the room. I have the urge to fall. If it were open, I know I would jump. I am going to crawl out of my skin. I'm bending over her. I see why she is bleeding. Her tongue is being bitten through.

I jam my hand into her mouth and start to scream. I am bleeding. Now the nurse comes. We are tearing at each other like lions, my mother and I. I push myself up. I have to get out of here, just for a moment. I push the nurse onto the bed. I am feeling along the walls for the door. The room is flickering in and out of my view. I can hear my mother's left arm hitting her face again and again, turning her nose black and blue. I think I will go mad.

Run into the hallway now. I can make out the shapes of the nurses by the counter. There is no noise. The hall is empty. There were only three nurses that night. I can hear my mother grunting. In her room, her leg kicks up in the air around her.

I know that in a moment I will fall. I try to get down low, but I don't know the way. I need to crawl to where the nurse is standing. I see them move toward me. I reach and find a collar as I go down, down. There are people running past me. It is the resident. Then blackness.

I wake up on the hospital floor, arms wound around the nurse's legs. I am screaming while waking, then blackness again. Shivering consciousness, nausea, and dead legged. I try to drag my way back home along the walls. I can hear my mother's breath. Hear it like I heard it as a child, warm on my cheek as she lay down with me, whispering promises she couldn't keep.

Down again and the nurse is bent above me. I am grabbing her legs. I think she is my mother, and I'm telling her to wake up. I lost my mother once when I was a child. I left her in a store and walked off holding the coat of another woman. The woman took my wrist and ripped my hand off her coat, and I looked up to find a stranger's face.

The nurse pours ice-cold water on me from a Dixie cup. Patients are crying in their rooms. I can hear them. The nurse is pouring water on me again, and I slam the cup out of her hand as far and as fast as I can. I am knockdown running back to where my mother is.

The resident is there, along with others. The room is full of strangers standing, poised like stuffed grizzly bears, and my mother is still eating up her tongue.

They take needles from their white coats, drawing curtains on the screaming Haitian woman. She is reaching for me. She is pleading. I think I know what she is saying.

They are pulling me away from the room. This is the moment of our death, my mother's and mine, with an army of grizzly bears between us, whitewashed monsters with needle hands and number eyes, counting, measuring, timing, pulling me off.

Clutch the walls. Can't stand straight. The blackness comes again, rolling up from the ground of my vision, and I am falling blind, again. And I give in. Let me crash down here where it makes most sense. But the bastards run to catch me as I'm falling through their hands, their legs, then all of space. Patients call from inside their rooms. All are frightened. Everyone is drugged, dying. Only misery lives here.

I saw her as they were wheeling her out on the gurney. Finally she had been sedated. They told me it was a seizure and that seizures were common after brain surgery. The aide said she had been seizing too long. There was a possibility that she would have brain damage. Then, in a flash of white, the doctors, the nurses are gone.

My father had arrived after it had stopped and missed the image that was now burned into my brain of my mother's body destroying itself. When he arrived we did not move toward each other. We did not even touch. He rushed into a huddle with the doctor. And I was struck by the image of these two men describing what neither of them had actually seen. The doctor was explaining what would happen next, and I stood beyond their little circle interjecting, *Why was this allowed to last so long?* My dad shot me a look, but by the time his eyes reached mine, the anger had dissolved into exhaustion. He was like a dog waiting for someone he knew would not return. And these words filled my head as if they had been spoken by some strange, distant voice: *the first part of her is gone.*

I went to collect her things from the room—her book and glasses on the nightstand . . . the bathrobe smelled of her. There was blood on the floor, on the table. The woman with bone cancer pulled herself up from her bed, grunting once with a deep pain. She got down on her knees on the floor to help me collect my mother's things.

To stop my mother from seizing, they gave her enough Ativan to keep her almost completely unresponsive for days. She could barely speak or open her eyes for almost a week.

Once again, they put my mother in the ICU. I knew my father wasn't going to stay. He looked exhausted. I didn't even ask him to. He called to me as I walked away, that I should come home to rest. I couldn't rest.

My mother and I used to swim out into lakes and seas together. We lost ourselves in the streets of foreign cities, following a train of thought for hours, losing our way so happily. When we returned, Dad would sometimes be upset. Where had we been? He had been worried. More and more over the years he joked, *I feel left out. You are leaving me out.*

I slept on the waiting room couch. Like a fool I tried again to sit with her, pushing my chair back against the wall so the curtain hid me. But they found me, and I was banished once more to the waiting room.

The waiting room was two thick doors and a hallway from the ICU. There were others there with relatives in the ICU. None of us were friendly, yet all of us were comfortable with one another. None of us were polite, and yet all of us were helping, bringing coffees when we stepped out, waking one another when we overslept. Extreme pain makes shorthand between strangers.

The Italian family slept on the couch across from mine. Mother, father, and daughter curled up together beneath an unzipped sleeping bag. We all ate from the snack machine, staring at the white wall above each other's head.

My sisters called me often at the hospital promising me that they would be back. I knew that they felt guilty and that they really shouldn't. This was not their mother. This was not exactly their responsibility.

I stayed those nights knowing that that is what my mother would have done. It helped to imagine she was I and I was she. To become her was to have a mother again. She had shown me how to be with someone who was dying. I had watched her with my grandmother Easter. I had watched her with my babysitter Liz, who while living with us received a diagnosis of terminal lung cancer in her fifties. My mother cared for them both. I stood at eleven and twelve years old in the doorway to their rooms uncertain. But she would usher me in, put me to work. And I found that I liked caring for them dying, that of all the places in the world I could have run to try to escape my fear, the only solace lay there in the dying room. There was magic in the final days and a sort of ecstatic feeling in the final hours of life.

The veins on Easter's hands were purple-green coloring the skin draped thinly over. My mother put Easter's hand in mine. Easter's breath began to stutter and then knock against her chest like a drum. *She was waiting for you*, my mother said. And then Easter was dead, her hand slowly cooling, her face slowly setting, and the nurse removed the plastic mask and wiped the white froth from her lips. My mother cut a lock of hair and put it in my pocket.

I was not with Liz when she died, and this was right. She and my mother were meant to spend those last moments alone. My mother told the story when I came in the morning. I sat down next to Liz. I didn't want to touch her hand that was four hours cold. Her lids were slightly up and her eyes snapped to my direction. *She isn't dead!* The nurse explained it was just reflexes, but those eyes stayed on me.

My mother told me how she had pressed a wet cloth to Liz's face throughout the night. And how Liz had had a dream that my mom was floating over her in flowers, wreathed, orange and purple flowers that were growing from her head.

Lying in the waiting room I wonder whether Liz's dream was in truth a vision. And this is my mother's blooming.

The Italian family's other daughter had a tumor that was strangling her esophagus. She was younger than me and lay in the room next to my mother's, sucking on ice cubes and crying.

In the waiting room, under my pillow, I kept my mother's travel clock. She had attached her name to it, written in ballpoint on white tape probably stuck there sometime in the eighties. My mother kept everything until it died twice and ran off to bury itself, and then she kept the maimed, broken remains. Her *waste not want not* farm girl upbringing made her frugal to the point of almost madness.

One of her closets was a bloody battlefield of gadget parts. The main bodies were gone, blown up—only shrapnel and limbs were left. She died before she found their matches, and still I cannot throw them away. I know I've seen the missing parts somewhere in this house, in this life. I think I see them every day, the missing bits. My life is a blur of short-term memory loss. It's like the game where you match head to body to feet, but it doesn't make sense as a whole, and I always have that eerie feeling that I've just missed the chance to fit it all together for once—all of it—objects, ideas, life. I'm one degree from making it all match, and I will die that way.

In the ICU my mother was very busy for a woman who was hardly responsive. Speech therapists, physical therapists, occupational therapists would try to coax her to open her eyes. She would slowly work the lids up, exposing eyes that seemed dead, that stared blankly, accustomed to the blackness beneath. I wonder now what she saw under those lids when they clamped down on her for days on end, locking her into internal landscapes where all the colors, the roads, all the skylines and water lines, the visitors, thoughts, emotions, were hers.

The therapist would ask that she lift her arm, and slowly she would drag it through the air above her head. Sometimes she would moan, and it came like water from her mouth, with the odd word struggling to stay afloat. The words, on their own, opened a doorway, each one leading to something that seemed recognizable, and yet I couldn't be sure at all times what she wanted to say. I tried to complete the ideas for her. I looked for any sign of recognition. But she never responded. And then would come another word, kicking violently to stay above the low gargle, and my mother would pound a fist in exasperation on the iron railing of her bed.

I remember being frightened that she would never wake up. The residents barely had time for my questions. They were so rudimentary, I guess.

Ms. Butler, they would say, *your mother is resting safely.*

But will she wake up? Will she be the same?

Ms. Butler, your mother is fine.

Well, what do you promise me? Give me specifics.

Ms. Butler, she is not out of the woods.

Well, what does that mean? What are the dangers?

Ms. Butler, lack of oxygen to the brain can be serious.

I am grabbing at their coats now. I am searching for them in all that white.

They seem to say, *Patience, Ms. Butler, is a virtue.* And their pockets are beeping and they are gone.

Her main doctor comes and speaks with my father. They pat each other on the back. *Well, you are the best,* my father says. *Well, you deserve the best. After everything you've given to this hospital,* the doctor says. At least my mother is lucky, loved by a man with influence here. He casts a special glow around her bed. The Italian family watches the exchange between these two men. They hold their daughter's hand.

I waited days in the ICU. I worried that my mother would wake up stupid, that the lack of oxygen during her seizure had caused damage to her brain. After giving her the Ativan, they had taken her down for an MRI, but we still had not received the results.

She was still and moaning for so long. Her eyes seemed dead when I held them open. But there was one thing that gave me hope—when she would walk her fingers along the bed rail. It reminded me of a game we played when I was little. She would walk her fingers up my arm until she reached my neck and tickle me.

I lay a hand down, just beyond her moving fingers. There is a look of humorous concentration on her face until she finds my hand. The eyes circle around under the lids. I begin to see that when I speak, she always responds. She gives a low moan, a wolf's howl. The doctors say, *Ms. Butler, she is not out of the woods.*

Well then, I think, we are in the woods together, calling out to one another. The moon throws us light. She lifts her arm. She starts to grumble.

I hear my name. The word stands alone even in water. It is rooted to the bottom of the sea and springs up, cutting through the sky. It is what I climb to find her.

My mother is smiling. Her eyes race back and forth beneath the lid. I sit on the edge of the bed. Her arm is plugged into the wall, and all the chords are pulled straight as she reaches out. The arm drags itself up over my head and around my neck, and I am pulled to her, right against her cheek, and she is moving as if she wants to speak, mumbling many things I cannot make out but already know.

Slowly she woke up, and finally they moved her to the rehabilitation ward. On her first night there, we lay, two in a hospital bed, illuminated by the city lights against the window. I saw the silhouette of her face—eyes open in the darkness.

I think we'll have to name my tumor, she said, *and it will have to be a diminutive, of course. Let's make it sound like an angry child, like a nickname for a little boy.*

We called it Chester. And for the next sixteen months I would remind her of that name. She would forget it, and I would remind her, and she'd say, *Ah yes, Chester, my angry son, my second born, my derelict. If I survive this,* she would say, *I want another baby. I'll give it a nice name.* This was the kind of thing she would say that let me know she had woken up changed.

My mother used to tell me a story about us. We were not like others. We were better. And worse. The world in which we lived was not designed for us. She warned me before I started kindergarten that I might have trouble in school. She did not want me to get upset. She said that I had a brain like hers—flawed but special. As she filled my head with this, all those early childhood years, I had no idea who she really was. It was as if another child were talking to me instead of the accomplished woman that she was.

She never had truly close friendships. She had moved too much. She had reinvented herself too many times. The friendships of her childhood were rendered anecdotal, living relics of another life, another woman.

She stayed in touch with them to support, to reminisce, but never to confide. Close friends see you at your worst, but hers would draw a blank face as to what my mother's worst was. Realness was too fragile a position for her. For her friends she was caregiver, big sister, even mother.

I have a photograph of her holding a baby doll. The doll is almost the same size as she. In this image she is captured, never a finished child—never a finished woman.

Irene had named her after Myrna Loy, a popular actress from the thirties and forties. Myrna Loy was as far from the rural Midwest as my grandma Irene would ever get.

In the little town of Wykoff, my mother lived surrounded by a large extended family, all staunch members of the local Missouri Synod Lutheran Church. This denomination teaches a literal interpretation of the Bible, including creationism and a belief that only people who have faith in Jesus will go to heaven. Everyone else—irrespective of any good they do or how they live—is on the road to hell. It is a harsh doctrine, and she began questioning it at quite a young age.

When she went off to college, she began to learn about other religions and to meet people from different cultures. And slowly she let go a little more of her Lutheran roots. Still, no matter how many years she put between herself and her childhood or how much worldly knowledge she acquired, she never was able to completely shake off the fear of hell that had been planted deep within her psyche.

Whenever she was in a semiconscious state during her illness, those fears would come rolling back in. She would become obsessed with the idea that her family would try to bring her back into the fold. My mother had her own beliefs and they were private, almost secret. It was hard even for me to get her to open up.

I wake up in the middle of the night to a line of light shooting out from the door cracked open to the bathroom. That's what I always used to say as a child—please leave the door cracked open. I hated the dark, and when my mother got sick, I hated the door. I would have taken it right off its hinges if she would have let me, but she wanted to feel independent.

I see her through the crack, coming to open the door in her white nightgown. Instead she slams the door shut. She is confused, she is sick. I can hear her coughing, full throated, and when I open the door, she is feeling along the floor for the toilet. It is her first reaction to treatment. I sit behind her with my arms around her waist so that she doesn't sink to one side as she is prone to do these days. I remember seeing her reflection in the toilet water, the pained expression on her face, and I had to look away.

My mother built a universe for me as a child. A place she ruled over like a goddess from my picture book of Greek myths. But now something was dragging her out of that world. I still see our faces reflecting in the water of the toilet, hers in anguished heaving. Mine was quick and pale before I turn away.

I lay in her bed with her that night, and she tried to be a mother and I tried to be a girl. But we were like two people who had fallen out of love—suddenly bereft of all that had been magic. She told me she was absolutely certain that everything was going to work out. I told her I was certain of the same. Then silenced and exhausted by the effort of the lie, we lay side by side, mouths up like two fish in a boat. I watched the darkness in her bedroom curl; shadows turn to us like pointed fingers. This was a place that she had told me about. This was Irene's view into the fall.

As a child she was good at everything. She could run fast, throw far, hit home runs, turn cartwheels, and dive over the entire tumbling team. She could turn double flips on a trampoline.

Every day she would help her father in the fields. She could drive the tractor, shoot a gun, and trap gophers for ten cents apiece. She would cut off the tails and pin them to her belt for later proof of her bounty. When my mother was small, she was sometimes recruited to use her little hands to pull baby pigs from a sow's birth canal when the birth was going wrong, and she once adopted a struggling lamb, setting her alarm clock to get up every couple hours through the night to give him a bottle.

In a photograph my mother's dog, Skippy, stands balancing with her paws on the tops of two chairs. Skippy looks suspended in midflight. Little Diane and Cousin Judy sit on the chairs so that they do not topple over.

My mother stands in front, arms outstretched, grinning ear to ear at her stupendous achievement.

Little sister Diane believed that my mother, five years older, possessed magical powers. My mother would sometimes taunt her, *Bet you can't get down to the dining room without using the stairs.* Diane was flummoxed. My mother lined her feet up on the baseboard that ran the length of the stairs and surfed all the way to the first floor without touching one step. When she reached the bottom, she whipped around triumphant—*bet you didn't know that trick!*

Sometimes it was hard for Diane to have a big sister who liked to trick and tease her, a sister who was always first at whatever she did and forced Diane to stay on her half of the room that had been delineated by an actual line of chalk. Yet Diane always knew that she could count on my mother to be there when it really mattered. One day Diane's beloved cat, Torny, went missing. My mother helped Diane search the fields for three days. They found the kitty dead, probably struck by lightning, partially decomposed. Diane could not bear to touch her pet, but my mother scooped the remains up and helped Diane give Torny a proper funeral in their ever-expanding pet cemetery.

Mom had read every library book in the one-room schoolhouse they attended—all two rows of them—and then she had read them all again. She had read the Bible from cover to cover and memorized many passages from it. She and Diane checked out books in a neighboring town, where they went every Saturday to take piano lessons. On one of these Saturdays they made a discovery: a basement that was full of old books in an abandoned schoolhouse down the road. The two little girls set out to retrieve them.

Tall grass had grown up around the schoolhouse, all the paint was peeling off, and snakes lay en masse sunning themselves in the window wells. My mother yanked open the rotting cellar door and climbed down into the spooky basement. Without reading the titles, she went tossing them up to Diane until they had reached the amount they could carry. They lugged their prizes home and laid them out in the sun to kill the moldy smell. This was how they discovered Pyle's *King Arthur*, Plutarch's *Lives*, and *Little Women*—all stamped Fillmore County School District 76. And this was what led Diane to realize my mother was her Jo March.

When my mother got sick, she would mistakenly call me Diane even more often than she always had. I would get so angry, and she would say that Diane had been her first little girl. In her first months of illness, Diane and I watched my mother try to change the course of her disease. *Bet you can't get down to the dining room without using the stairs.* There was that old twinkle in her eye, that old belief that she was magic. But all the tricks she had perfected—they no longer worked.

In her heart she was as she had always been, the sleeker, faster version of herself. She still saw herself that way. So why had dates on the calendar begun to dance? How did buttons and doorknobs not work? And walls jump in her path and cupboards crash on her out of nowhere, and numbers go jumping around, refusing to work together to add themselves up?

She cried every day. She asked me if I thought she was failing. I didn't know how to comfort someone who could do that to herself at a time like this. My mother never gave herself a goddamn inch. Cancer was a mistake she had made. All the things that were happening to her body were happening because she had not yet found the trick. She had not yet found the key out of this new cage.

A million times she promised me that she would get us out of this. I will be there when you have children. I'm gonna get so old that you will want to kill me. Wait and see. You ain't seen nothin' yet. I'm tougher than you know. She swore all this to herself and to me. These are promises that mortals make.

With my mother's illness, there was born this new shorthand in my family, a shorthand for the shorthand that had been. Despite how difficult this was, the family felt closer, and we saw each other far more often, especially as my mother grew worse. It felt sometimes as if my sisters had moved in with us, even when they were back in Maryland and D.C., it felt like they had just stepped out for a minute because we spoke so often on the phone.

Hold on, Al, let me pull my pants up.

Hurry up, Cindy. She's calling to me.

What do you think it is?

I don't know. Her nail beds suddenly turned blue, and her hands are swelling up. She keeps forgetting where she is.

I began to live on the phone with my sisters and they started to come almost every weekend. They would alternate. They must have told me a million times to take a break, to get away. I didn't hear them. My mother could not take breaks. And so neither could I. This was a mistake. I would have been better for my mother in the long run if I had paced myself.

I was twenty-three then twenty-four with just a job, no career, no idea what to do or how to go about it. I had exited the real world where my friends were living on like normal people.

I felt passion about nothing. Failed relationships cued up behind me. Some of them overlapped—I wasn't loyal. I spoke on the phone with one ex-boyfriend. He had rekindled with me, but now he said he couldn't do it. He knew I wouldn't stay, and he didn't want to put himself through all of it again. He left me with these words:

I am a person from your past. I hope someday you will find some meaning in your life, Alex. Everybody thinks that they are special. And then they grow up.

A shot went off in me and I hung up. I felt sad but relieved he had taken back his offer. Most things were no longer worth the fight. When I was eighteen and less had happened to me, I chased complication. I had time for difficult people, thinking I could crack them on my knee. Thinking I could reach some kind of secret center that I had envisioned. But people like that were not worth the effort. Let them be somebody else's tears. I was done collecting broken things.

I had met someone right when my mother got sick. I cancelled our first date the night that she was diagnosed. He came to visit us in the rehabilitation ward after that first seizure. I lit a candle before he came in to clear the smell of hospital. I washed my mother's face and combed her hair as if she were going on a date. He wore a suit because he worked at the Frick. I could barely look him in the eye, he was so handsome. He ate my mother's hospital food to make her laugh. She told him right then and there she loved him.

My whole relationship with him took place in my mother's house. Six days out of seven, he stayed nights with me. A couple months in, he said the apartment was starting to get to him. When I had 4:00 A.M. nightmares, he would hold me in his arms and he would cry too. I liked to make him cry. I liked having a witness. Nobody could see him except me. Five days out of seven, I told him he could not come until 9:00 at night. He started in collecting resentments. I had no room for it. I would melt onto the floor, and he would give in. I was not being manipulative. I just could not see beyond her. *You'll go crazy*, he said, *go ahead and make yourself crazy.*

He used to describe the view from the kitchen window. I've always loved that view. It reminds me of the film *Rear Window*, but he called it the alley of his discontent.

I'm not sure what happened or in what order it happened. I'm sure that I was sorry. We both had our faults, and who cares to count when there is such an obvious circumstance to point at. I lived for the small things, but he didn't. He wanted trips to California. He wanted sleepovers in Brooklyn. Brooklyn felt as far as California. I had to be near her.

In the end, we lost. At the start, he would wake up and sing me Gram Parsons's "Brass Buttons." We were like infants in August, always smiling, always staring. We did well with falling. And for a little while, how little else there was. He delivered me; who knows where I'd have ended up without him at that time. In the end, I hurt him, but he would forgive me.

I tried again with someone else several months later. I turned a friend into a boyfriend hoping he could lead me back to my old life. We went to the White Horse Tavern in the middle of the day. The air was that green just before rain, and as we opened the cab doors, it came drumming on the windows. He had a way of furrowing his brow as if he needed me to translate every thought I had into his language. I liked this and I hated it. Our first dates were our last. After a month he said a bunch of words that I'm not sure he had had time to organize. He called it off. I begged him to reconsider. He called a couple of days later, and we resumed the friendship, but it sputtered out. We'd messed it up.

I made Cindy cry over the phone. *You have to believe that you are good enough*, she said. But I knew I was turning into someone else, a person who had little to offer. I was twenty-four and living at home, a stupid job. A loser. I could see no future. I imagined that I was the daughter my parents' friends would shake their heads at, *That one got away, that one was lost. Didn't take after either of her parents. They are so accomplished.* The world had shrunk down to my strange, contorted mother. My terrain was the house I had grown up in, now old and shabby and filled with so much sadness.

I think she found in me the only person she could trust. She was the most trustworthy person in the world, but she trusted no one. She felt that her own deepest problems and concerns were her solo business. She did not discuss them even with her closest friends, and all her relationships were built on her taking care of the other person.

Many of her stories about her past were filled with a kind of palpable loneliness.

Growing up she took solace in being with her father. He never questioned her about religion. He accepted her as she was. He was proud of her and loved her unconditionally. She said that when she ran to find him outside, he looked to her like a spring chicken flapping his arms against the sun. She would run to him for comfort when she was in trouble with her mother, and without saying anything he would lift his wing and shelter her beneath it. That is how she always remembered her father. He was her spring chicken.

Her dad never got an education, didn't even attend high school, but he imparted his philosophy of life to her through his strong work ethic and unfailing optimism. He was one of those people for whom the glass is always half full—a genial gambler who outbid his hand when playing cards—and often won. His commonsense sayings became legendary in the family: "If you don't want to get fat, don't eat so much" and "Why do you want to get so tall? Most of the work is down here on the ground."

She watched him rise early every day to milk the cows and work the fields. Being lazy was the worst thing he could say about anybody, and nobody ever accused him of that—even in old age. He was a good husband who loved his wife, and my mother said they had a partnership that she admired. My mother idealized her father. She imbued his silences with wisdom. He was loving and warm, and she often said she wished she could find a man like that—implying that my dad was not that man.

She was the first person in her family to finish high school and go on to college on a full scholarship. She told me of her struggle freshman year having come out of a one-room schoolhouse in a tiny town. Her teacher had done the best he could with a class that ranged in age from four to eighteen.

Her dorm mate was the only other farm girl at college. Together they stood out in their homemade clothes. My mother said she was a social outcast who did not go to dances or to parties. To catch up academically she often stayed up all night to study. She described nights where she forced herself to stand by an open window so the cold air would keep her up. These stories did not feel like the typical clichéd parental tale of struggle. They were not so easily discarded as my father's jokes about having walked ten miles barefoot in the snow. I could feel her torment in these stories, a loneliness that still hung over her.

There was a pond in the woods outside her dorm where she would walk when she was upset. She would walk around the water until she had stopped crying. She was terrified that she would lose her scholarship and be sent back.

Four years later she graduated Phi Beta Kappa from the University of Minnesota, named its top sociology student. She won a full scholarship to pursue her master's in social work at Columbia University, where she would eventually receive her Ph.D. Yet so many years and achievements later her concept of herself had not improved. And her sense that she never quite belonged remained.

She told me I was a visitor from some other place. She told me it was her responsibility to keep my celestial destiny intact. There were some very abstract pep talks when I was a child. She would promise me to protect my spirit. She believed her spirit had been crushed.

People always felt she truly saw them. She was the favorite aunt, the favorite cousin, and the trusted confidant. She could become consumed by other people's needs, giving hours of her day, months of her life to helping someone. I watched her become impromptu estate planner for a dying friend, or act as someone's ad hoc immigration lawyer. She stayed extremely close with her first husband's little sisters, whom she had helped through the death of their mother at a young age. Apparently Irene had been like this. She was the first person at someone's house after a death or birth, lending support and cooking meals.

My mother befriended a homeless man whom she saw break up a fight in the middle of the street. He would come by every three weeks for his "allowance." She would stand at his corner with him and chat. Every Christmas he would bring us presents, a bronze angel for my mother, a pair of silver earrings for me, and once, inexplicably, a full-length velvet skirt. Their relationship spanned more than twenty years. She worried that his HIV would take him; he was diabetic, going blind. But Leon would outlive both my parents.

I would bump into him eight years later, downtown one hundred blocks from my home. He was completely blind, shrunken on a corner. I asked him if he remembered my mother. He seemed taken aback. *Of course I do. Who was she again?* By then I was wondering the same.

When she finally came home from the hospital it was September. All of us were poised. We were told she could be dead as soon as three months away. Every day I worked to pull her out of a depression, coaxing her backward from the deep, from beneath a veil of gloom that threatened to swallow her whole. My father was gone more often than not at this time. And my mother was swallowing me whole as I smothered her.

Every morning in September I would walk her to the corner of Eighty-sixth Street for a donut. She struggled all along the five blocks, the cancer and the treatment playing a tug-of-war for her, exhausting her so that she had to stop and sit several times on every block.

We had a bench we always went to in the park, and she would eat her donut there beneath a giant tree, this lady tree showing off her frock of turning leaves. My mother did not seem to truly grasp her diagnosis. I didn't know if the damage to her brain was what impelled her not to see what she had coming. Or was it just me—the mere presence of me—that kept her from admitting she could die. She had promised me once as a small child that she would not die until I was ready. She thought it was a surefire thing—her arrival at white hair, bent back, rocking chair, her settling slowly into old age and then her slipping, effortlessly, away.

She could not hold both the coffee and donut at one time, so we switched off. We were becoming a combination person in September. It now took two bodies to do the job of one. I learned to think like her, to anticipate her needs so she wouldn't notice how much she really needed help. If she thought that she could still do everything, she would be happy—or at least happier. I thought if I moved quickly enough, with an embrace, with a napkin, with a gentle push through a closing door that I could keep her happy.

I shadowed her, catching crumbs or coffee drips. I read her face, her mouth when it wanted more, when not. I read thirst, frustration, fear, and exhaustion. I stood agape at the foot of my mother, the woman of my life, as if at the foot of a mountain waiting for something to come down.

Aunt Diane came to stay with us. She dropped out of graduate school and worked on the book she was writing only in pockets of time throughout the day. Most of the time, if she wasn't with my mom, she was researching glioblastoma on the Internet, holding her face up close to the screen, jotting down notes, clicking the keys, pulling the chair in closer, then pushing it back, rising and pacing and sitting again.

My mother had always described Diane as a sort of Joan of Arc. I could see that in her now. She was poised for battle. She called me into the closet in November, shut the door on my sleeping mother, and said, *There are no silver bullets, Alexandra.* She had been looking, searching the Internet for some kind of alternative, some kind of medievalesque drip that could wrench our lady free and draw her back into our world.

There are no silver bullets, I repeated, as if I hadn't known that, as if I didn't know what the words meant. I hadn't yet grasped that death was actually equal to death. What was about to happen to my mother was as incomprehensible to me as trying to define the color blue without using the color to define it.

We sat in the closet together as if we'd been told for the first time that we would lose her. We crouched in the closet like two children. It felt impossible that there were no silver bullets for the woman who had been a silver bullet. We made a pact then without even speaking that we were her guards waiting on each side of her until death came. Diane's devotion to her at this time was the purest love I had ever seen. All the complex dynamics between them completely disappeared. I forgot that they existed. She put my mother first with every breath.

Mom started sleeping in every day—something she had never done before. She said she didn't want to open her eyes, that in dreams she had gone back to the days before all of it, to sixty-six years of living before dying. My aunt and I would lie with her. In the morning she cried. She spoke about leaving Dad and me. We would have big discussions then, my aunt, my mother, and I. Most of them were about her family.

She spent November thinking. She seemed to be growing angry with her family. She knew they would be coming soon to save her soul, and she made me promise I would protect her. Diane would answer the phone and say a name, and many times my mother just shook her head, too overwhelmed by thinking of what her family was thinking. She said they knew how she had left the church and religion behind. She was sure that they believed that she would burn in hell. My mother pulled the covers to her eyes when the phone rang, closing her lids down on the day, and waited stone silent as Diane would answer, carefully, protectively, holding my mother's hand.

In our morning conversations we covered ground, roamed for miles, for years, over time, stringing her life together, weaving narratives and combing out knots, pulling apart fears strand by strand in our circle of three, ironing memories and patting her hands, cursing the ones that deserved cursing, making her laugh—and then we'd make breakfast. This was our routine every morning.

Invariably, we joked and guffawed through breakfast and followed it by placing a gigantic sweet—a cinnamon roll or a big cookie—in her hands. Invariably we decided against her showering, and invariably she showered. Then she would try to do all the things that she had done before she became sick. She could not accept that she had permanently lost some of her abilities, and so I watched her push herself every day as if she could overcome brain damage through dogged, mind-bending effort.

She set up a desk in the living room so that she could look out the window. She sat there making notes about notes, trying to outsmart her new mind. She followed a growing trail of paper in a chase that felt new to her every time. Her life had become defined by trying to perform tasks she was no longer capable of. The thing about glioblastoma is that it kept from her what she had lost. A ruined brain does not know it is ruined.

I would wander in as if I had been passing by instead of watching her from behind the door. The tilt of her back was a stage. It showed the shifting of sorrows within, the daily surrender to her new, feeble mind, the confusion to which she was condemned.

I would wander in and lay my hands on her with hope, with such desperate heartache, and a feeling of being adrift in an ocean of ice-cold and indifferent water. We were two tiny specks of shit without even our dreams to sustain us.

She would feel my hands and say, *Your father is probably going to get on my back really soon about writing that book with him. So don't expect me to have as much time to futz around with you, Alexandra. You don't know what writing a book is.*

A sob comes different ways. It can start at your heels and go rising up, curling like a wave when it reaches your mind. You start to swallow sorrow, breathe it in and out like air, it fills your lungs and stops your heart. You draw your arms around her wanting so much to push the health in, heal the cancer, or to drain the life out of her if nothing can be done. Sometimes you think that you would kill her if you had the heart. You just want to save her, to heal her with that surge of immeasurable energy, with that sob before it crashes one final time and rolls away, leaving you dry and numb.

The steroids that controlled the swelling in my mother's brain also made her manic. She was positively effervescent at times—a flurry of Socrates and Tony Robbins's style lines. She was far more prone to monologues than conversation. It was as if ideas were stacked up in her mind, in a long line, like dominoes. She would simply take off into a gust of effusive speech, her eyes, her thoughts ever expanding, like the wide wings of a great, long bird, imparting ideas and philosophies as they flew though her mind. They would float down, one by one, until the last thought would stop her, and she would fall silent, abandoned by her own digressions and suddenly, excessively fragile.

She decided that brain cancer was the perfect excuse to take time off from work and organize her house. So she pulled everything out of the closets at once and laid it all out on the hallway floor. She would carry the small objects around on trays to ask what we wanted to save and what we could dispose of.

Objets d'art, objets d'art she would call as she came padding along, a slightly drunken maitre d'. The hallway was filled with old furniture, paintings, rugs, shoes, blankets, clothes, and a million little objects such as gerbil wheels. The sprawl staged a coup and spread like an army through the length of the house, consuming the carpets with clutter. It was as if there were holes in our house, in our lives, and the past was pouring in on us, water filling up a ship that was in the act of sinking. We walked with care—my mother especially, calling out when something crunched underneath her feet. Crying out when a glass slipped from her hand and crashed into many tiny pieces.

She would cry then but not let us help her. *I have everything under control,* she would yell. And what could we say? She always had. We couldn't rob her of that feeling now. And so we continued, letting the house fill in, watching my mother pace, and trying not to bother her with our concerns. We reached out for one another from across the rooms, laughing behind frustration from what had become of our lives. We all laughed a great deal together, waiting until we were alone to cry.

The items from my mother's closet of gadgets required the most sorting. The boxes held labels like "watch parts," "staplers," "travel cases," "hot water bottle caps," "flip-flops," "flashlights," and "homeless plastic parts."

I watched my mother for several days while she roamed around the house, hovering by different piles. She was pulling out and piling up at a much faster rate than she was sorting. She would never finish what she started and kept moving on to the next pile, becoming more and more confused and more exhausted.

One morning I found her at the kitchen table. She couldn't admit how overwhelmed she was. She had built her life around her ability to organize herself into oblivion. She had built her life around the belief that anything could be achieved if she worked hard enough.

I think about the way she lost her ability to organize data and numbers in her head and remember dates. She found the concept of time so elusive now. We had begun to give her an extra hour before appointments, and even then she rarely arrived on time.

She was seeing doctors often. They monitored her treatment and the progression of her illness. She was receiving the obligatory chemotherapy and radiation that we were told would probably not work but which would allow her to become part of a clinical trial at the National Institutes of Health. The trial was promising within limits. She was excited, she said, *to be a happy lab rat out there on the frontiers of science.*

It was as if her brain would become caught, entangled in something. I would see her strung up, as if in a tree of thoughts. She would stop whatever it was she was doing. While dressing she might get caught in the act of rummaging through her sock drawer. She would lift a pair out and put it back into the drawer, over and over.

Our front hallway filled up with the contents of our closets. At the end of every day, I would clear a path through the center so my dad could come home. I watched her try to do it by herself, her hair in her eyes. Her broad back, her farm hands as she called them, grasping at some small ashtray or object. She would think about a pile and move it around but then leave it and the next day alter it in some way.

I started to clean through the piles one night after she'd gone to sleep. I slipped away and began to wrap things in tissue paper and load them in boxes. It didn't matter if it all went away. We didn't need any of it, so I packed almost all of it and carted it away. In a day I had finished it all. I couldn't stop myself. I wanted it gone. My mother was angry at first. Then she admitted that she felt grateful, and then she forgot it.

I can finally laugh when I think of her cleaning the house. I can finally laugh when I think of her. *Objets d'art*, as she called them. *What, may I ask, is this objet d'art?* she said, holding the dog collar that I wore in high school. She comes back to me sometimes to laugh. She comes back and holds my hand to sift through memories and make them less sad.

She had always hated the concept of the holiday letter. This year was different. She wrote one for her family in Minnesota. The letter read like a contract. It functioned like a contract. She seemed to believe that if she wrote it now and mailed it in December, at Christmas she would be there when everyone received it. She did not wait to start. In October she had already begun to write a little of the letter every day while she stooped over her desk at the living room window. She left some spaces blank so she could fill in her diagnosis—as if it were continually changing.

She was pushing herself to be active. She paced between her file cabinets and the desk she'd set up in the living room, papers in hand. She started a portable filing system that she could lug around with her so she wouldn't forget what she was doing. She was like a human tackboard with Post-its and pens fastened to it. Notes on her hand that showed her what she was doing right this moment.

In the letter she spoke of her hopes for improvement after radiation treatment. She was due to receive her next MRI in December, and she hoped that the results would be better than those of her last. Presently, things were not good. She had two new tumor sites. One of the tumors was growing along her thalamus, she explained in her letter, and the other was growing along the line between her occipital and temporal lobes. Both tumors had grown from nothing to the size of a finger and a walnut, respectively, in a span of four weeks. She explained her diagnosis a thousand times over the phone to friends and relatives, and I would hear her try to comfort them. She was trying to be certain, just as certain as she had always been, that if she worked hard enough, she could come through for us all. She could win.

My mother's tumors, left untreated, could kill her within weeks. That is what the doctor told me. After her return home from the hospital in late August, my mother started several projects. Each day she gave a little time to each. Most of them she would never finish.

Before she was sick, my mother finished everything. Sometimes I think it was the neurological impairments that kept her from completing projects, but then I think she also understood the importance of having something to do each day—the importance of having little reasons to keep going when the big reason was so evasive.

With tumors holding court in your brain, a wide-open day is not a pleasure. You don't live for long-winded leisure. You live for purpose. You live from one activity to the next, from one distraction to the next. My mother believed that through the systematic application of her mind to tasks, she could prolong her life.

The blank spaces in her holiday letter were surrounded by words of rallying. All the terrible things the doctor had said, the things that she must have remembered, sounded better and more hopeful when she said them. She used the words of someone trying to sell an idea to the world, but most of all to herself. The outcome of her letter wouldn't depend on the diagnosis she was given in December. In her head the final outcome was unquestioned.

Many days I thought could be her last. I thought she would die or cease to be herself entirely. Yet every time I thought this, she always came back, and each time it was less of a relief.

We might be talking in our new, simple way, and then all at once the old her was speaking, nuanced and astute, awakening in me a frantic child who was dying for its mother. And then just as quickly she was gone.

Throughout that fall she left in pieces. She would talk nonsense one morning, then return, but each time a little more of her stayed back, as if she were being carried away bone by bone.

She resisted death, and I continued to pretend that I believed she could survive. We played a game together, each laying down a lie. We offered ourselves at the foot of the other's image. She was invincible. And so was I. I was taking her disease in stride. None if it was so out of the ordinary. That was a favorite phrase of hers during fall. My mother thrust forth this idea with an iron hand—none of this was out of the ordinary. And certainly we were not allowed to be angry, because we were lucky, had been lucky in general in our lives. Anger was to be avoided at all costs.

We lived in a world taut as a cave striking matches against the darkness. We let matches burn down to our fingers until the pain made us blow them out. We struck another and another and another—happily, as if we liked the heat, as if the darkness were a normal thing.

I became more frightened. I began to lie very still inside my life, knowing no wishes, having no dreams, hating and loving her only. I could think of nothing else and no one else. Youth stopped sending invitations. My presence was no longer required. I caught glimpses of people my age moving around, engaged in life, changing away from me.

My connection to my own life strained. My best friend had gone off for graduate school in London. I tried to see people every week at least once, but these meetings felt to me like dispatches from war. Friends were supportive, but I didn't ask for much. I needed to feel like I seemed strong. I was afraid that if I asked for too much they would reject me. I begrudged them their happiness, their lives. I felt tremendous self-pity, and maybe to combat that feeling I came to believe that I had been chosen to go on this deep spiritual pilgrimage to help my mother die. I staggered between those two places. I was as low as I was uplifted, as miserable as I felt enlightened.

As my friends went forward, dancing, they looked like a million clock hands, now faster, faster, while I only watched. The world and youth can have each other, my mother and I said, but it was just myself speaking. She would never have said that. She wouldn't like my standing alone. Well, she had lost her ability to see what was happening to me.

When she was sick, my mother never pointed to the distance between us. She allowed me to believe that I was with her, and she was not alone. I thought that I could take her right up to the edge of life and hold her hand as she made her way across. But there is a distance that my eye could not see. Only the eyes of the dying see the road they are following to leave us.

From the moment she was diagnosed, my mother was alone, and for all my insistence upon staying by her side, I never left the spot where she began. Though I wanted to know, and to see, I never did. There is a human resistance that kicks into gear when nearing the presence of death. The resistance in the mind is so strong that I wonder whether we create it or it is created completely outside us. It places a veil over the eyes.

By November our protective intentions were starting to look more like controlling behavior. When the closets were clean, my mother decided to redecorate. *My bedroom lamps date back to your father's first wife,* she said.

She had the couches reupholstered and the windows recurtained. She was planning a new bathroom floor when my father started worrying about her spending. She didn't seem to be thinking of money. It didn't concern her as it once had. He tried to reason with her, and she exploded. She couldn't believe he didn't trust her and that he would turn on her like this. She had always handled the money—she had always made decisions for the house. She said he was being disloyal, and in a way he knew she was right. He apologized, he acquiesced, but secretly he had the estimates forwarded to him. She never knew.

It was already easy to infantilize her, to pull the wool over her eyes *for her own good.* That was what we said, what we believed. I look back on that time and see her like a caged thing trying to run as she always had. I see my father and me reining her in, and I wish I could go back and let her go. That broad, strong thing she'd always been, I'd let her disappear into the distance, running until she was out of sight.

From the beginning of her illness, we were extremely careful. We thought we were such experts. We made lists: always close dishwasher, make sure the corners of all the doors are padded. My father and I could not accept the fact that we were fated to watch her be hurt, and that there was nothing we could do to truly protect her. She was going to slam down on the floor like a tree. She was going to cut herself open. She was going to seize so hard that she couldn't speak for days. We couldn't catch her every time. We suspected that from the beginning, and so we honed in on the little things. We were like insects buzzing around her, making her crazy.

I like to think that she was walking in and out of the next world when she was sick, the scenery around her was changing, and that is why she would crash into things, slam into doors and cut her forehead against cupboards.

It hurt me to watch her turn shades of black and blue that would take months to heal. But had I imagined that she was undergoing invisible system changes, making paths between two worlds, maybe I could have let her be. She would be walking in one place and be transferred to another too fast to clear her path of impending dangers. It was selfish of me, because she wanted to fall. She would rather that than lose her freedom.

For sixteen months, she was our hostage. People told my father and me to let her go. They said she needed dignity. I shouldn't hover as I did. It was humiliating. They didn't have to see her walk into walls or trip over the edges of rugs every day because she dragged her left foot behind her. They didn't see her silk scarf go up in flames from a candle, which she didn't even notice until I pulled it from her screaming and stamping upon it on the floor.

I insisted on sitting outside her shower so as to stop her from falling. She wanted to shower alone. Sometimes she would bang her fists against the tiles and cry for a moment. Then I would cry. Then she would comfort me. I wondered who the patient was.

In the end, after all my efforts, she was gone, beaten down by the disease. Back when they were sewing her head up, they had told me she would die. They had handed me a page of words. I drew on the page like a child. I tore it up, I never made a single change, just covered up the thing I'd always known. Even at the start I could accept that she would die. Yet I never could accept the fact that she would suffer.

My mother chose to cope with cancer by trying to remember who she was before it. She tried to remember what it was that she fought for — that life that she no longer had. That person she had once been, possessed of so much ability, the woman on all her ID cards.

The Red Cross continued to call long after she had become sick. She was a first responder. Once there was a fire, once a plane crash. She would pack her bag. I tried to tell her that she couldn't go, but I would stutter. This woman was my mother. My father tried to tell her, but she unleashed a torrent of words at him over the phone.

You are both ridiculous, she said. *You are the ones with the brain damage.*

We left her alone. Maybe she would tire herself out. I stood in the doorway.

She pulled herself out of bed and made her way to the bathroom in short intervals — bed to chair, chair to couch, couch to doorknob. Her hands could not grip the brush so well. I took it from her hand, righted it, and passed it back to her. *I think my hair is growing back, don't you?*

Yes, it looks wonderful.

I think it will be back in no time.

I think her hair will never grow back. It's been five months, and nothing has changed on the bald spot where she was radiated. She is out of breath. I help her to the bed.

Bring me my socks, please, and also some pants and some underwear.

Do you want a shirt, Mom?

Of course, dummy. I think those people have been through enough already.

She worked so hard to be the person she always had been. She didn't notice many of the errors that she made while attempting to fulfill these roles, but then all at once, something would happen that would grab her attention and would break her heart.

I came home one day and she was sitting in the living room, her nightgown half on. She had much difficulty dressing. Apraxia is the inability to manipulate your own body.

She would put her arm through the head hole of her nightgown without understanding what was wrong.

Then I noticed smoke coming from the kitchen. In the oven I found the dinner she had tried to make. I had asked her a thousand times before not to cook without me. She thought I was being utterly ridiculous.

Alex, you can't crowd me. I don't know how to do things anymore because you won't let me. Besides, I'm going away soon to visit my family, and I don't want you to come.

I came back into the living room and said nothing. She had the faintest smile. I asked her what she was thinking.

I am planning how I will get out of this. You are going to be proud of me.

I asked if she wanted me to help her to her bedroom. She told me not to move her. She didn't want to forget the plan that she was making.

I have to focus because if something were to happen to me, you and your dad would not survive. You would be at each other's throats. Where is my holiday letter? I need to finish it.

At her desk by the living room window, she spent a week transcribing her address book on a Rolodex in giant marker so that she could make out every number. But the numbers kept moving. They danced around the page, she said. Nine times out of ten she couldn't dial a number right. She couldn't add a line of figures up or count out a handful of bills. She didn't know the name of the street that we lived on.

When she cried, she wouldn't leave her desk. She wouldn't stop working, and the papers became wet, the words and numbers smudged and ran together. I began just to sit with her. After about three hours, exhausted and frustrated, she would go to her bed, and I would lie down with her. For several months, this was our daily schedule.

I dreamt of her around that time. It was her corpse I spoke with in the dream. She was seated at a table at the end of the earth, attempting to write a paper or something of that nature. I recall her eyes, how grief-stricken they were, and her purple skin. She seemed not to notice me. I wondered whether this was hell. Is this the fear her family gave me? Now I dream of my dead mother trying desperately to perform the tasks of life, somewhere alone and cold; I cannot reach her to help her.

She was a psychotherapist. Though she advised them of her new circumstance, most of her patients continued to call.

Her practice specialty was male CEOs, but she also had a range of clients, male and female adults of all ages. I think what attracted her to psychotherapy was the same thing that attracted her to social work: she longed to understand how people coped with the vicissitudes of life. And I think she also found that the strongest part of who she was would come alive when she was helping other people in ways she could not always help herself.

I was worried at the beginning of her illness about what it was like for her clients. Were they just humoring her, or was she able to tap into some magical reserve—that stronger self in which she had always taken comfort?

I had had to make the appointments because she couldn't match up date to time in her schedule book. Numbers and time frames, dates and appointments were in constant flux in her head. Each day there were so many bits and pieces of things in her mind that she couldn't make sense of it all. She might have a Tuesday the seventeenth in there somewhere and a 2:00 P.M. She would come guiltily tapping at my door. *Tuesday the seventeenth*, she would say with outstretched arms, completely baffled. Most of the time I would tell her. I hope that I helped her most of the time. I think that I did. I remember that I did, but some of the time I know that I bristled, and she knew it. She knew what she had become—a burden. I was tired. I couldn't stand it after a while—her repetitive questions. I would give anything to go back and wait on her again.

But when her patients called for their sessions, I would watch her after I handed her the phone. It was ludicrous and yet so natural, though you would have bet your life a moment earlier it was impossible—my mother could interpret her old self.

It was a self I knew she no longer understood. She might as well have been playing someone else. She was no longer the person she had been. Parts of her brain were dead, so parts of her had lain down. They didn't see the sense in moving. Parts of her had been laid bare, others submerged like land under water, like thoughts under cancer, like brain beneath tumors that built sticky roads through the inner landscape.

Yet every time a patient called, she nailed down just who she had been to them. She played out like a tape-recorded message. I'm sure they felt a change, but it didn't seem to be the drastic, humiliating trauma that I had expected. Only my family and I were given access to the new her. With the rest of the world, she could and she would rally.

I would linger a moment outside her office door and listen to her voice change in response to the gentle coaxing of formality. I would kneel in the corner, listening for sounds of the mother I remembered. I wanted so much to run in there to sit closer as she spoke.

During her illness, if I heard her laughter in another room, I would stop to listen. In Central Park I always chuckle at the squirrels stopped suddenly by something—a noise or smell—their little front paws curled up against their bodies, their eyes wide and waiting, picking up something on the breeze. This is how I was when she laughed. I was frozen. I learned quickly to savor the moments. I began to savor her right off, probably even the first day that I went to that doctor's office to pick her up. I kissed her good-bye a million times. I studied her—the way she moved and spoke. The way her hands looked. But the voice is what moved me, what moves me still.

When I would sit at the door and listen, my mother's laughter made it seem like not quite everything had been taken from her. She came back when she laughed, riding a note in her voice like a comet. I could pick up the scent of time open-ended and lazy, like plans, like weeks that you think will unfold without end.

What have you done with my things? she kept repeating. *I know that you stole them.* She would come at me like that—angry and untrusting, and that is around the time I stopped pretending to be perfect, the selfless caregiver, and the anger started to take over me by December.

I was consumed by her disease and by the anger at not having the mother I needed to turn to especially now. I lashed out in tones I would regret—no longer able to call on a reserve of patience. Once as she was accusing me of hiding her favorite pants I became so enraged I yelled out that she was a piece of shit. *A piece of shit?* I don't know where that language even came from. She cried for a great part of two days. Even as I sat with her apologizing profusely she was inconsolable. *I feel like a piece of shit,* she said. I wanted us both to die, just go to sleep.

The constant fear, the stress of mind and body, the heartache had rotted my composure, and I became a beast attempting to play human. I felt like a domesticated wolf. I had to excuse myself to run, to howl, to hunt distraction, and then I would return to her, my tail between my legs, my sharp teeth hidden in a clenched jaw, praying that I could bring her through this without tearing her to shreds.

Every errand that she made me run, every time we sat in her office for me to assist her with some project—it all felt like she was playing a cruel joke, or I was, or someone was, offstage, an evil devil trying to exhaust us beyond any limit we could survive.

Sometimes I would collapse in hysterics, having left her in her wheelchair in aisle three of Bed, Bath and Beyond. It felt like we were trying to run errands in the movie *Memento*. Here I was daily humoring a crazy woman—a mad hatter trying to find my way with the Cheshire Cat's map. I wondered seriously whether she was torturing me, setting up situations heartbreaking and horrible to both of us. I longed to be woken from this, my mother shaking me with her beautiful strong shoulders, the old her, ringing that bell in her voice box telling me to get out of bed.

We went to Minnesota. We flew on a chartered jet supplied by a generous family member so that she would not get the flu. Her immune system was depressed from the radiation and drugs she had been given.

It seemed as if we saw every family member. They all made time to see my mom—they gathered around her. They were warm and kind and discreet in the face of how drastically she had already changed.

My mother's family had always been exceptionally gifted at caring for their old and their unwell. They were inclusive and devoted and seemed to know exactly what to do and what to say to keep her confident and happy.

It was an epiphany for me to realize that my mother's greatest strength, her ability to care for other people, was reflected throughout her original community. I realized I had never quite seen anything like this, a town that was an extended family that took responsibility without question for every member.

And yet my father and I did not leave her side. We wanted to make sure there would be no talk of God. She was in a wheelchair for most of the trip, though she would get up and walk about the house with someone's help. He and I were never far behind, listening to be sure that nothing was said that would upset her. There was one cousin, a self-selected shaman who we worried was trying to start a conversation. However, in the end, he did nothing more than recollect sweet and affectionate memories with her, and she was charmed by his presence. It turned out to be a wonderful trip.

At her brother Donald's house there was an old Super 8 recording of her jumping on a trampoline in her high school gym. The image sputters in black and white. There are ripples in the film as she jumps up and down, up and down, forever.

In another shot, she is part of a human pyramid. She is smiling out from her place at the front doing the splits with a stack of high school girls behind her.

She couldn't get down the basement steps to watch the video. We finally carried her, but she still couldn't see. The tumor had blinded so much of her vision that she couldn't make out the details in the grainy film. I walked forward until we were inches from the image projected on the recreation-room wall. Her face was tilted sideways as she tried to locate herself. She still had sight on her right side, but she was standing too close. The image of her jumped up and down over her strained expression. She kept saying, *I can't find myself. I can't find myself.*

In the first autumn of her illness, my father was always traveling for work. Conversations with my mother that fall could still be devastating. There was this daily process she went through from despair to euphoria and back. To be with her was to feel this horrendous terror. She was still herself. Her voice and her affect had not changed. She still had a mind that was powerful enough to rake over the reality of what was occurring.

Sometime in the late winter, everything about her would go flat. That is when she began to speak in simple terms, and I would be left to imagine that her words were metaphors for things I longed to hear her say.

In the years since, I have come to accept that any magic in the words was affixed there by me. These were simply blunted thoughts from a broken brain. It was my desire that weaved the myth of some remaining meaningful connection.

But in the early days, the early weeks of her disease she was still our mother. It was out of character that my dad had not assumed the worst when she had experienced those first few symptoms. He was the sort to warn you that an earache left untreated might become a brain infection.

It was a source of humor in our family. He was a worst-case-scenario kind of guy, and as a child I was painfully aware of the terrible fate that could await me during a bike or boat ride or climbing a tree or riding on skis or roller skates. She made fun of him for his anxiety—a good thing that would help him lighten up when he became too morose. She said his alter egos often woke her in the morning, reporting to her from behind the pages of the *New York Times*. She named these alter egos Dr. Ominous, Dr. Deplore, and Dr. Lament. Thanks to these three men, before she even made it out of the bed in the morning, she knew exactly what man- and womankind were up against. It must have been unthinkable to him that his young wife could be taken first.

In those early days, as we waited for her diagnosis, my father could be found in the chair next to her bed, silent then sobbing then silent on and off throughout the day. I had not yet met the man that I would marry. Though I thought I did, I did not understand how deep the love of a partner could run. On her first night in the hospital he insisted on staying alone with her.

I imagine that they were up late into the night planning their battle out like soldiers. I imagine they made promises they would be forced to break. They told me the next morning they had counted their blessings, a new childlike nightly tradition they maintained.

In those early days, my father played the hero. He began calling her his bride, and she gave him such fanfare. It killed me. It made me feel revulsion. I knew about their unfinished business. She had wept to me about my father all my life. I knew he was no hero. Now I was unable to fall for his white knight or for her damsel in distress. It saddens me that I could not take comfort at the time in my parents' drawing close together. I understand now that I was competitive with him.

There seemed to be floating this idea from them both that while the rest of us were fretting, my father was doing. He was planning his bashful bride's next month, her next six months, and all of eternity. My father was so well connected in the medical world that both he and she believed that he could save her. Surely there was some new secret and radical treatment out there somewhere. He traveled to the edges of the earth via speed dial—top doctors from across the world. As with all things that he did, he threw himself into the task of saving my mother's life. Between his phone calls and research and strategizing, he was also managing with work. He was off to his nonprofit to run the thing one-handed for a spell before he came galloping back to kiss my mother's hand. But the days marched over us like a procession and one by one his phone calls were returned and each hope extinguished. And her white knight began a slow and pathetic slide right off the backside of his horse.

I don't remember if it was a moment or whether it was over the course of several weeks that our gentleman began to take his leave. It may have been around the time of her seizure. My memory of him begins to fade right around then. That was when the traveling for work seemed to set in.

At the time I saw him as cruel and questioned whether he loved us at all. I was young and rigid because of that. I could not wrap my head around what it was he was going through. I thought this man who could be so brave out in the big world could be brave in this tight and airless space where we lived now. But those are two distinct types of bravery. I did not realize I was stronger. If I had I might have made it easier for him. I might have reached out across my suffering to his.

In a thousand ways both giant and small he left her alone in her agony. I tried to be her husband, to sit by her side at the absolute edge of her existence. Part of me felt entitled to be there—more entitled than my father. Another me longed for the white knight too.

At first she made excuses for him. He had huge demands on him at work. But the space he left beside her grew more and more grotesque the more distorted and contorted her disease rendered her mind and body.

She started to ask me about him constantly. She started to pit me against him. She wanted to know where he was at every second. She began to tell me things that I had heard before, though in far less devastating versions. Now she said he had broken her heart, ruined her life, stolen her work, wasted her talents. She told me that if this was how he responded at a time like this, then he had never loved her.

I called my sisters, crying. I think they were torn. They were angry with our dad for running, but they were also worried for his health and heartbroken for him. They would plead with him to be more present. They were, after all, not strangers to this, our father pulling away in times of pain. When he would respond to them with his denial and his well-formed excuses, they would turn their focus onto me. They would offer their help. They would try to fill in for our father.

I believed what I had always believed as her confidant, that she was his victim. I had to defend her both from him and from the world, and now from death.

Call your father. Tell him that if he does not come home in twenty minutes he will not see me again.

Dad would come home, and I would greet him like a pit bull. He would dodge my bite with anger, then with sympathy. He would attempt to be my father. And then when it would not take came the leash.

Do you comprehend what this is costing? I am drowning. I have to make money so she can get care. I need you to contribute in the way that you are able. Your mother's mind is no longer working. She is struggling with her own brain. You have to be wiser and smarter than she is. You are twenty-four years old, no longer a child. When I was twenty-four years old, I was already a father.

He was right. I should have been ready to take them both under my wing. I should have a respectable, high-paying job. Instead I was a spoiled and soft, ill-prepared little rich girl and now was my comeuppance. My parents' thinking themselves invincible had let me dream—let me dream too long—and here we were. Neither one of them could keep the illusion alive any longer. This was the "real life" they had so often told me about. The real life they had lived but I had never lived. I was terrified, and yet a part of me had been hungering for this. This was my chance to make my way.

My father continued to be gone. Gone even when he was at home. As gracefully as old men doing tai chi in the park, he moved through the motions of father and of husband right there next to us, yet he never made contact. He did for us but he could not feel for us, he could not be. I let him go. I let my need for a father go.

Our friendship dissolved. All those horror stories I had heard about my father from my mother and sisters—they came knocking back. Now I understood and felt a new emotion for him, something like total abandonment—something that felt very close to hatred.

Each day her anger and disappointment grew. It seemed she was consumed by regret, by sorrow and her anguish about her life with him. We clung more and more to one another. I found comfort at least in being able to be there for her. This was the abandonment that she had always feared. She was no longer useful, no longer in the role of the caregiver, and so she was abandoned.

One morning she told me that she was leaving. Unable to even leave the building by herself, she decided she would rent her own apartment. *All the years I put up with his shit, write this book—write it faster!* She made me research assisted-living homes.

If he cannot be here for me now, then our marriage was a lie, she said. I was numb. I helped her compare and contrast highlighted details of these homes. I took a tour. Sometimes I imagined this was my office job, personal assistant to someone basically a stranger. Sometimes that was what helped me concentrate on the tasks at hand.

Those long-term resentments she had held against my father, which in better times she had processed in a complex way, were now simple and base and utterly devastating. Something I had always understood as my mother's sadness, ancient, unsolvable, was now showing itself to have always been hell-bent anger. She was burning it all down, every lovely word that she had spoken to me, every philosophy of life, every wonderful story of our family, the very world she had laid out for me. She was burning it down.

Sometimes I would lie in bed at night and recall us. We were happy once. We had quarreled and hurt and disappointed one another, but I know we were happy. She loved him. I know she loved him and believed in him and he the same. It had not been a lie. And this was not a lie. All of it was based on something real, but it had become so horribly distorted, a mania born of misery. I wondered whether it was worse to have them here but gone. I felt orphaned, left with two automatons. My mother said Dad had left his family once. He could do it again.

She transferred some of her financial accounts into my name. She accused my father, saying she did not trust him to give me the money she intended for me. She made him swear to my face that he would give the rest of the money she was unable to transfer. My father and I could barely look at one another. There was a shame in the room, and I did not know whom it belonged to. It was in all of us. In that moment I realized we had completely come apart, ceased to be ourselves, all my memories of us, my very sense of who we were as individuals and a family—it all felt like fiction.

Dad had always been anxious about money, but this was so dark a place for us to have arrived. He touched his hand against his cheek. He closed his eyes. He promised her. He walked out of the room. I felt no pity for him. I was blown out and hollow, and nothing felt real enough to feel any way about.

Then sometime in winter her anger disappeared. I don't know if it was gradual or sudden. We were dealing with somebody else, a third someone else, another iteration. This woman just wanted comfort, a foot rub, a warm body next to her in bed. This woman wasn't clear on the details of what had been going on. The few times that I cried in front of this woman, I received a weak pat on the shoulder. The kind of pat a stranger would give. She spoke in clichés. *Suck it up. Nobody said it would be easy.* This changeling, sometimes I wanted to shake her. I imagined candy rolling out. She was as authentic to me as a piñata. She wore strange, bloated flesh, a sunken facsimile of my mother's body. This one did not have to forgive my father. He was a pleasant man who drifted in and out. This one did not have to let me go. I was no more her child than someone on the street. She was nice, this new generic, loving, putting her arm around me, patting my head as if I were her freckle-faced neighbor. A cat that doesn't know you will let you pet it as it passes by because that feels good.

She did not grieve and she had no regrets. Slow and stupid and strangely content, that's how she was. This new person was the result of both the progression of her illness, the damage to her brain, and the effects of the medication for her treatment. She puttered around in her own mind like a daft floral-covered housewife. And yet at the same time she was imbued with a new and divine light. She was genderless, asexual, a charming, rotund, cherubic being. I responded to her as I would to a giant toddler, tickled by her little observations. I kissed her sausage fingers that looked like they would burst, her cheeks like roses from the steroid treatment winding its venom through her muscles.

She delighted in the smallest things, the little rewards that had become a program for her days. We kept a gigantic box of Godiva chocolates in her medicine closet. She called them her vitamins. I liked to watch her eat them. She would suck away, float to another place, overwhelmed as a dog is by a biscuit each time at the richness of the thing. A faint smile would spread across her face. *Are you going? Okay. Did you just get here? Okay. Okay. Okay. Okay.*

I sat with her. I held her hand. The new flat affect in her speech and body made her seem sarcastic and droll, though she was the opposite. She was utterly unapologetic. One might even say that she was the happiest I had ever seen her. The puerility that had possessed her was ingenious, as if a sweet angel had taken pity on us and showered her with an opium dust. I sat with her. I kissed her hand. The fat green vein on her left hand was still the same, a mark left from another life.

Now she had one thought where she had once had ten. And she thought one way about each thing in life. My mother had been put out of her misery, put down. Her black wave of sorrow had discontinued crashing and receded, into a thick and salty sea in which she now bobbed like a buoy, her face painted on.

And one day after many weeks of this woman greeting him always and only with a smile, the gentleman finally came home. To his extinguished flame. There was only love coming from her. He seemed to be what she remembered best. She held his face as if she had birthed him. At the edge of her bed my father would sit rubbing her feet, and she would praise him. Sometimes he would hang his head and cry.

This time I lingered at a distance, watching them as if they were a painting. These two nubs of people had reemerged. I began my first miniscule fluttering away. Life no longer lay with these two people. Life was something that waited beyond this—empty words, but at least they were there in my head.

Every year my parents were invited to give lectures at a health spa in Arizona called Canyon Ranch. They would lecture on topics related to healthy aging. It was a gorgeous place in the middle of the desert, and my parents would stay a week or two and enjoy the spa. Every morning they would do a sunrise walk, although this year my father went on the walk alone. Even though she could not take part in many of her usual activities, my mother wanted to go, and we all knew the fresh air and sunlight would make her happy. Her doctors were fine with her traveling, especially because there were doctors on staff at Canyon Ranch in the event that anything occurred—another seizure, for example.

My mother told me she planned to give a lecture. I was nervous and I told Dad that we should stop her. He became very angry. He said it would be wrong to tell her now. This was who she was and fuck the audience. He was right, of course, but at the time he made me angry. I was so obsessed with protecting her name, as if she could be blamed for her condition. I remembered seeing my parents' old friend Betty Friedan give a speech after she had had a stroke and how much it broke my heart to see her struggle for her words, the painful pauses. I saw her as a victim. She was not a victim. She was doing what she loved to do. I didn't get that.

My mother was excited and relaxed. I had never seen her so relaxed; usually she was nervous. But it was so painful for me at the time. I wanted to hide her. I could only think the old mother was calling to me to protect her name. But the old her would have let the new her speak.

My father had become a different person around her. He seemed to have accepted who she was. He was not embarrassed. He was proud of her. He seemed to take great solace in taking her arm, in leading her through the world with him. She rested her head on his shoulder. He had become her number one. I was relieved.

On the day of the lecture my father went first and was, as always, charming and wonderful and natural up there. My mother was seated alone in the right front row. I had come in late, and to avoid crossing the room during my father's speech, I sat down in the left front row next to a woman and her husband.

It was late winter, almost eight months since she had become sick. She was more swollen then ever from the steroids. The hair growth on her scalp was patchy, some of it was curly, some of it was straight—apparently this can happen after radiation. There was an asymmetrical bald spot with a thick incision scar running down the center.

Her pink wool hat had an elastic band that fastened right under her chin (her idea). Otherwise, the hat would slide up on her bald spot and sit like a cone at the top of her head. She looked like an absentminded elf. *Ridiculous,* I thought. She had become so pragmatic in her dress. She had asked for little fasteners to attach her gloves onto her sweater, the ones I swore off in the first grade. She thought they were great. She was surviving. I cared. I wanted my beautiful mom, the statuesque, the elegant—the bright and witty one that everybody fell in love with. People had always envied me her. People had always wanted to keep a piece of her for themselves. She was all mine. I loved that feeling, of having people covet the woman that made me.

But I do not know how I could not have been proud of this other woman. This amazing one who didn't give a shit, who attached her gloves and hat and plowed her way through hell and back each day with shaky steps. This was a magnificent someone, statuesque in spirit, majestic in her heart, but my vanity, my pride, my fear of the world's rejection of her—it blinded me.

Her clothes always had spots on them now. She was messy now. I didn't always have the energy to keep her clean. When I thought of her as something that was funny, I would push it down. I didn't want to see her that way. It wasn't right to have these thoughts about your mother, to want to cry and end up laughing. It was all so gruesomely funny at times—those moments when friends and family were at their most solemn faced, and I wanted to shout out, after choking back laughter. It wasn't just for her that I was working to keep a brave face but for them. I had become a person who never stopped performing.

Tonight she had dessert on her shirt. I was disgusted with whoever had allowed her to bring in that ice cream from the restaurant. If she had been a child, they would have had the decency to ask her mother. That's what they didn't understand. Her motor skills were those of a one-year-old, and her concern, her ability to notice when she stained her shirt was almost nonexistent. My mother's friends should have learned how to clean her up after a meal. This would have been more helpful than all the phone numbers for me to call and talk things through.

The waiter at the spa restaurant had been kind enough to give her a plastic container of chocolate sauce so that she could pour it on herself. People are so thoughtless in their thoughtfulness. In the conference hall from my row on the other side of the room, I could hear her breathing. It was deafening these days. She poured the chocolate sauce down the front of her shirt on the way to her ice cream. It dribbled over the ice cream onto her pants and pooled on the rug at her feet.

The woman to my right took notice and rolled her eyes at me in a confiding manner. I had so many emotions running through me that I simply did not know how to respond. Then she started going all out—nudging her husband and whispering, *Who is that woman?* She shook her head not only at me but also at the people in the row behind her. Her head went turning on its neck, sending the judgment out into the room, to all the rows, looking to receive whatever she could back as if conducting her own cruel and silent auction.

At least my mother was oblivious. Her vision was contained within the elastic bands of her hat. Her mind was married to that ice cream. The state of her brain was such that a bowl of ice cream seemed to transport her to another world entirely. I felt as if I were watching a show on nature. The cameras from far off had zoomed in on her burrowed somewhere in a vast forest, no predators in sight. There was my tiny, ratty mother working her way through a golden nut. Her strange childlike self, her fat belly that had once been flat was poking out from under that filthy shirt.

The woman's face turned back to me, distorted and hideous, the head shaking back and forth. The woman's nails were shining in the overhead light of the conference room, her body stamped down on the chair. Her husband was obviously successful enough for her to maintain that perfect body. She probably had little else to do. Before they opened their mouths, I knew they hailed from the South. She had that major hair and nails. She looked like a well-shellacked sorority sister.

When the man asked my father a question, it was too much to bear—to see my father smile at him. Dad did not know what was going on. He was too busy doing his thing up there. And I thought to myself—is this really how her life will end, with the world scoffing at her? With the world applauding her husband, her writing partner—the man who said so often these days that without her, he couldn't write as well, would do nothing as well? Was this her fate, after so many years of being a social worker, of studying and defending the rights of older women—women who had reached an age she would never reach?

I would never see her old. She would melt like wax right where she was, still desperately trying to grow like a flower in an oven. The petals go first and then in a moment she is gone.

My father stood at the podium, this time like every other time, the very image of a relaxed genius. He was where meandering and focus rendezvous—a duet so perfected after so many years it had become a careless talent. There was always something about Dad that drew everyone in, different from my mother, who seemed to always have a psychic understanding of who you were.

With Dad it was his confidence even more than intelligence—his utter lack of doubt and then that very faint whiff of unapologetic fragility—that made the rows of seated listeners lean in. Sometimes it seems to me as if they worshipped him, all of them, including the woman now pouring chocolate on herself. I love my father. I feel good on his arm. I feel good when people look at me and see my father. And I hate him. I hate that I think I cannot be him, will never be as valuable as he is, will never be as loved.

My mother had once stood shining at his side; now no one in the room would even guess they were together. They think Dr. Lewis did not come. I wanted him to jump down from that podium and take her in his arms.

She woke up one morning and told me we had to go to the bank right away. She needed to go through the safety deposit box. She couldn't remember what was in there. *If I die, I don't want you and your sisters getting into it over what belongs to whom.*

We arrived at 3:30 and the room containing the safety deposit boxes was closed. I told her I would bring her back tomorrow. Using the wall to hold herself up, she yanked her hand from mine and began making her way over to the teller's window.

There was no one in sight. She pressed the buzzer before laying her head down on the marble ledge to rest. The teller came and stated once again that the room was closed for the day. My mother lifted her head from the ledge. Her face was dry, but her body seemed to convulse with sobs, her hand became a fist, and she rapped on the glass again. Both the teller and I didn't move. Standing where she'd left me at the wall, I was so tired. I was always so angry in winter. I wanted her to die. I wanted to die.

I know that I walked over and put my arms around her. I remember her weight falling against me. I remember the feel of her soft, fallen-muscle, tired flesh. She had grown heavy. I could barely hold her up. I swallowed winter with my anger, swallowed whole days to keep from yelling out. I was so desperate not to hurt her.

I travel back in my memory and want to lay my head against hers on that ledge and give her kind words. I wanted to be cradling her in my arms. But I wasn't. I was just holding stiff, mechanical me against her sunken frame.

She reared her head back and pulled herself up by her fists on the ledge.

I've no time left! I've no time left!

The teller pushed open the door to the safety deposit room. My mother straightened up then, clutching her cane, holding her purse as she always did now, by the end of its long strap, so that the bag dragged along the floor behind her. And when you asked if you could carry it, she would always shake her head.

She stood her cane against the desk and braced herself to sit down as the box was placed before her. She put her hands on it and pulled it against her. The teller stepped outside and closed the door. My mother's tears stopped as suddenly as they had started.

Get your notebook, honey. We've got work to do.

I decided I would take a class to get me out of the house. I decided on a grammar course at Instituto Cervantes. My goal was to learn Spanish grammar off the page. I had become fluent through osmosis during a year in Spain when I was eighteen, and I wanted to know the names of the tenses I used.

I envisioned myself on the other side of Manhattan, pounding out the mathematics of language like a mental kickboxer, but in the end I spent those eight classes talking to my teacher about my mom in Spanish. Twice I left because my mom was seizing. The third time the teacher urged that I stay. She said the fact that my mom was already in the emergency room with my father meant I could finish her class. I stayed, not because I agreed, but because I was beginning to give up on her and on my plan to save her life.

I had once thought that by doing little things I could save her life. I set alarm clocks, made notes. I abused measuring cups and spoons. I ranted if her noon medications were five minutes off. She called me Attila the Hun. I oversaw her physical therapy schedule, whether or not she was moving enough. I had taken charge of all these things because I did not trust anybody else to be as organized as me.

Before January I hadn't left the house for more than two hours' time with the exception of evenings while she slept next to my father. He helped her with late-night trips to the bathroom. I worried over them— my older father helping my heavy mom so late at night. I slept with one ear tuned to that door.

On those stolen nights I would splurge on a cab down FDR Drive and open the window. I would drink until I could speak openly and then whisper all of it to my friend Pollyne. She was the only one who never said I had to reclaim my life. Pollyne was living for her mom too. Her mom was chronically ill and dependent on her for financial survival. She had been doing it long before me, and she would continue long after I was free.

My mother had taught me a way of devotion. I knew that I would eventually fall below the heights to which she'd set the bar, but I vowed not to fall before my time. I promised not to break until I was really broken.

One day my Spanish grammar teacher told me of her aunt, who had lived for many years with Alzheimer's. A woman had cared for her whom they had loved very much. My teacher told me the woman's name; it was Myrna. It was a sign. Myrna is not a common name. That same day I phoned up Myrna Pedraza.

Once in October my dad tried to get a home health aide for my mom, and she had a fit. We heard about it for weeks. She insisted she could handle her life on her own, but she couldn't schedule an appointment on her own. Dates and times swam in her head. She would miss appointments and fall into depressions. Other days she couldn't line the toothpaste on the brush. She would cry because she didn't know why she had come into a room.

Brain stopped, she would say, staring. There'd been something she had wanted. How do you tell someone that they need help? How do you force assistance on them? How do you leave someone like that? Someone who only a few months ago was working emergency relief for the Red Cross, doing her taxes in a weekend, running the New York Marathon.

You don't leave someone like that. You readdress her letters in secret. You close faucets she leaves running, cupboards she leaves open, and pick her up when she falls like a kid in a sandbox but hurts herself more. You watch her get in bed, black and blue and deadened with frustration, two in the afternoon, to cry.

You signal her when she's rambling too long on someone's answering machine, repeating herself, asking you for the phone number to the house she has lived in for twenty-two years. You sit outside her office door like a deranged stage mother while she speaks with her old patients. Your hands clasped, digging your nails in your palms. *Please, God, let her get through this. Deliver her. Let her save face. How can forty years of hard work end in this humiliation?*

And she always nails it, and you race in to tell her. *Bad news, I've been spying. Good news, you've done it again.* And her patients keep making appointments. But it wears on you. The victories hurt because they remind you of what you have lost and what you will continue to lose—all of her—but for now her body goes on walking.

In February I realized that she was stuck, but not me. I could leave that house on my own and walk as far and as wide as I liked. I just hadn't. It was a strange feeling to realize I could leave. I should leave. Until then I hadn't had the strength to leave her, and now I couldn't find the strength to stay.

I gave it some thought and then I told her three things about Myrna Pedraza. One, her name was Myrna, an obvious sign, I explained. Two, she was described as nonintrusive, quiet, and three, she had worked as a "personal assistant" for another "professional woman" for many years. I wasn't against fibbing at this point. When I was little she cut my steak into tiny bits for me so it wouldn't look like steak. I felt that I was performing a similar service.

Maybe she bought it—more likely she knew that I was tired, felt I was edgy, and knew things were getting too hard for her. She could no longer convince herself as easily about her abilities. She acquiesced, surrendering that last dream of independence, and agreed to let a stranger into her house. I had what I wanted, but it didn't feel victorious. I knew that she had traded her freedom for my own, and that I had fallen below the bar. I had been broken.

In March I left her with Myrna—at first only twice a week, then three times, then four, then five and some nights. My mother didn't mind her at all. Myrna had a knack for being helpful yet invisible. She was an editor, putting her hand against doorframes to protect my mother's face as she passed, walking behind her, arms poised for catching, hands holding a trailing scarf like a maid of honor. I would see them sitting out in the park. Myrna Pedraza would wipe melted ice cream from my mother's face. They sat in the sun, Mom's eyes were closed and a faint smile on her face—always thankful for the smallest things.

I don't think I fully appreciated until now how easy she made things for me just by being her natural self. My mother never asked why this had happened to her. She always said why shouldn't it happen to me? She taught me that although seemingly random and indifferent to our human suffering, nature should always be respected and its intentions trusted.

Sometimes I think that the way she died was nature at its cruelest. On the other hand, I can flip the whole experience and think how poetic of nature to break down my mother's mind, to let me see how sleek and intricate it had once been. As she unraveled, she was revealed to me. Broken down unit by unit, my mother's brilliance seemed almost quantifiable. I began to see her brain as a map, and I was walking into that landscape. I was an astronaut and her brain, a planet. The topography was always changing. If I modeled it after earth and divided it as land and sea divide, then sections of every continent were being submerged bit by bit. You had to sit still and listen to her words; you had to watch her hands, the path that her eyes made, what she ate and whom she wanted to see that day.

I would stay stuck with her on one idea over several weeks until the thought that she had been thinking and rethinking changed before my eyes to something else equally nonsensical. My mother in crisis was something else. I believe all people are like this. Yet she was as true now as she had been before, it just took me a while to realize it, because she was so different. But this had been her all along. All her years of sadness had in truth been years of anger.

Our personalities are so complex, so varied, and carry in them so many elements that seem to be in opposition to each other. But I studied her as she peeled away and realized why she chose to stack one thing upon another. I understood why she left her anger at the bottom.

There were calm times and crying times as she broke down, as land became swallowed by water. Things that had once been connected were parted and sea channels born, connecting places that had once been apart. A new meticulous conversion of elements was constructed and then blown apart like particles of sand. These constructions were too detailed, the elements too tiny to ever be re-created. My mother was a death in progress. Every day didn't make sense but made perfect sense perhaps.

When people ask me what it was like, I say it was as though your head were a map of the world. Whole continents might be submerged. On second thought, that is too simple—it is more as if parts and chunks of continents were submerged. Families were split up, parents wailing for children, gardens divided row by row and across—flowers divided, petals divided and divided again. This was the extent of her neurological divide.

If people are like motherboards on a computer, if a soul encased in a body has a billion tiny plugs of possible communication to the outer world and other people, some of hers were unplugged. It was totally random. There was no pattern, no every other, no every third—no every hundredth. The changes in her were fleeting. One almost didn't see them. A sentence would begin like her and end as if someone else had said it—as if she had become tired in the middle and a stranger had resumed the work. I struggled to love this rewrite. God had switched the actress, the original formula was lost, the flower irreversibly divided.

In April I drove away from New York and from her, leaving her in the full care of Myrna Pedraza. My father said I couldn't take it anymore. I hadn't slept for days. I'd reached a record number of six. I was exhausted, but when I lay down at night, my body would rev up like an airplane engine, my cells would take flight, suspending me over my bed. It felt like I was holding my legs up, but when I looked, they were flat on the mattress.

There were nights when my bed would reject me, spit me off its face, and I'd shoot up running. I'd pace for hours to tire myself. City lights glowed outside the window. I knew that people were sleeping or living, and I could do neither.

I gave up and drove to Cindy's house in Maryland. Cindy had been begging me to come for months, but I hadn't. I always said I had to stay near Mom. Something could happen at any moment—a fall, a seizure, or a lost finger cut off by a knife. Worst of all, she would be sad, and I wouldn't be there. I imagined her staring out the window like a prisoner. I wanted to stay at that window with her. I couldn't. I didn't have the staying power. When she got sick she was chained to that window. It is a testament to the human spirit—the things that life will force us to endure, and the fact that we survive. If you had asked before all this happened if she could do it, she would never have said yes. As I drove into the night, I thought of how, at eighteen, I had left home and ventured out into the world, into my life. Months would go by when I wouldn't call her. I thought we had time.

As I drove I thought about all the lives I had once had that were far away now. I thought about being eighteen, about being twenty, about all the boys that I had loved. I felt like love was passing me right now. I'd turned my back on all that when she got sick. Maybe some of these cars held people that I would have loved. Fate had made me as pure as a nun. I had become a character in a novel, the spinster caretaker character. I was the one who gave up her life to cart the obese, lunatic parent around.

I remember approaching the Delaware Memorial Bridge as night fell. The sky was dark velvet, but you could see everything, all the details of the landscape rolled out. Water stretched on both sides, and trees looked like paintings on a canvas, creating the illusion of a big, round world. But there was no world out there. Not for me. My world hinged on a half-blind, bald woman who couldn't add or subtract, who couldn't remember her phone number, who couldn't cross the street by herself anymore. My world had been distilled down to nature's whim for a dying woman.

The person I had modeled myself after was going down. This is what happens to good people. So why be good? It was a free fall inside me. On the outside I was still five foot ten and twenty-five years old. On the inside I was thimble sized and falling, losing myself in that oversized suit of a body. I'd end up facedown at the bottom of my feet, and no one would be driving this body anymore. I would become a free agent, a feather, soulless, an aimless traveler with no call to put down roots, with no understanding of setting up shop on earth. I had no alliance. I wasn't for life, and I wasn't for death. I wasn't for me, and I wasn't for her anymore.

As I drove over the bridge, I cried. Seagulls circled over the bridge towers, and the air was wet and soft. I knew then that I had loved life once. I knew that I might love myself as much as I loved her, and that I could imagine wanting to save myself, to save my own life, but I wasn't there yet. Driving over the Memorial Bridge, I was not anywhere that I recognized.

Part of my reason for going to Maryland was to collect my mom's new dog. She had named it already, Emily, after Emily Brontë, her favorite writer. I was not looking forward to walking this dog. I had never had a dog. It was ridiculous that she wanted this now. She insisted that she would care for it. We wouldn't have to bother at all. She would walk it every day, she said. She needed an old dog like her Skippy, she said, the dog from the picture standing on the chairs. She wanted a puppy just like Skippy, and she told me she had found one.

I drove with Cindy to go pick it up. The breeders lived in a ranch house with framed painted portraits of poodles. There was a tunnel built out of their living room that ran into a fenced-in yard where the poodles could play. They were gun-toting, poodle-loving Marylanders. Emily was the last of the litter there. They said she did not like anyone who had come to look at her. Even the runt had found a home. But when my mother and Cindy had visited a month earlier, Emily had crawled right into Cindy's lap. Cindy had promised them that if they let Mom take her, Cindy would eventually take her if need be.

I looked down at the dog. She had big brown eyes with long eyelashes. She had red, curly hair. She looked like Red Fraggle. They said she was the biggest of the litter, had pushed the other puppies off the mother. I smiled down at her, though I did not feel much. I picked her up like a sack of groceries and stuck her in the back seat of the car. By the time we pulled up to Cindy's house, Emily was seated in my lap, her big brown eyes staring into mine with utter expectation.

Over the next few days at Cindy's I became slowly aware of the dog. She was a brat, but also charming. She constantly wanted to be held. She was pretty and she seemed to understand that. She had an extremely regal "sit." At night she would chirp and cry for hours to be let out of her crate. In the middle of the fourth night, I snuck down and took her out. She clung to me, lacing her paws around my arm. I took her upstairs and she curled up on my pillow, looking into my eyes until she fell asleep. *Fuck,* I remember thinking, *now I like her.*

I was supposed to leave that Sunday, but I decided to stay another week. Another Sunday and the same thing, a phone call home, the assurance of the two Myrnas that they were doing fine. My mother sounded relaxed, content. She would relay off what they had done that day; when she forgot, she would ask Myrna, and I would hear Myrna's gentle voice reminding her of their trip to the park. It was clear to me that Mom was getting better care than she had from me, at least in recent months. Myrna had managed to get her on a schedule. She was bathing, eating, going to the park every day, and Myrna was helping her run errands. My dad told me Myrna was amazing. He was very happy. And in the evenings he would come home early to spend time with his wife. I hung up the phone relieved that I could stay and yet still feeling somewhat guilty.

You have to stay, my father had said. *You need to get better.* Things had become really bad before I left. I had gone five days without sleeping. I was having frequent panic attacks. I had seen a psychiatrist, who prescribed antidepressants. I had resisted at first. My father was against them, but even he ended up begging me to try. I had started taking them at Cindy's house. I was so eager to feel different, and yet I could not imagine how these pills would change anything. Cindy had been dealing with my panic attacks. Sometimes I would wake her in the middle of the night and she would lie down in my bed with me as if I were still a little girl.

Sometime in the middle of the second week, Cindy told me that she could see me coming back. And I realized very slowly that I was. Each tiny step I took out of my depression almost erased for me the understanding of the step before. I noticed that I could finally sleep and that little things like walking Emily did not overwhelm me.

After three weeks I finally came home and found the house and my mom in perfect working order. Myrna Pedraza had taken over and everything was fine. *Oh, hi!* my mother said as if I had been gone for several hours. She was thrilled to see Emily, who dutifully jumped up on her bed. My mother had bought Emily a bunch of presents, which she presented to her as if she were a child. *This is my granddaughter,* she said smiling. I will never know for sure if she was aware of the meaning of those words or whether it was a kind of funny, offhand comment, or whether her needing a dog was actually her understanding that I needed something, in this case a new life to help me go on.

I was humbled by the effect Myrna Pedraza had had upon my mother. Mom was clean and bright, her every need seemed met. She spoke about herself and Myrna as a team. *Today we did this* and *we have been extremely busy* and *Myrna is fantastic with directions.* Myrna was so petite and slight I could not imagine how she held my mom up. She would be sitting smiling quietly in her chair in the corner. They did not seem to have that many conversations. They would coexist, no niceties, no manners per se, an almost psychic, intimate connection between a dying woman and her nurse. It was amazing to see. In my mind, Myrna became a kind of deity.

I could see, now that my brain was not fogged by a major depression, that so much of my clinging to the role of mom's caregiver had been about my ego. At least that was what it had become. I had wanted to be a martyr, but I could let that fantasy go.

My mother would play with Emily and brush her hair and fuss over her and yet she didn't seem to mind that Emily had become my dog. Though I tried to instruct her to stay with Mom, she followed me when I left the room. Mom began to sing "Mary Had a Little Lamb" quite often.

My mother had been wearing her thick Coke bottle glasses for the past two weeks. She could no longer put her contacts in. She would put a contact on her finger and move her hand right past her face. She could not find even the general area of her eyes. So I began to put them in for her each morning. She would praise and thank me. *I have the most wonderful daughter*, she would smile at Myrna Pedraza. It felt almost as if these were the good times, almost as if we had come back.

Doctors disagreed in June over whether the enhancements on her brain were necrosis (scar tissue from radiation) or new tumors. Her doctor in New York told her it was necrosis. She called me at work. I had returned to my dead-end job at Shadow Studios. I was happy to go back to that familiar place I had known before any of this happened. Inside those walls I could pretend that it was still that summer.

My mother called me at work. She said she wanted to be the first to tell me that it was necrosis. *INDY! INDY!* she yells into the phone. "INDY" is the acronym for "I'm Not Dead Yet." My mother had read an article about a fruit fly scientists had named INDY. They were manipulating its genes to make it live beyond its natural life span. In that fruit fly my mother found her own little Lance Armstrong.

I bring home a cake for celebrating. Both my parents are lying on top of their bed. *Oops*, they say, actually smiling. Her doctors are fighting. The one at NIH says no to necrosis. The one in New York insists. The doctors are talking among themselves. We are laughing at home. We convert tragedy into a comedy of errors now. We find everything hilarious. Most of the time my mother is in a good mood this summer. Maybe the weather, the sunshine, the plants and animals springing to life.

We are told the next day that it couldn't possibly be necrosis. The new enhancements have grown outside the area of her brain that was radiated. She called the whole family again to adjust the story. I pick up in secret from another room. I am sick of hearing her explain it as best she can in her convoluted way and of everyone's damn questions. My mother has grown accustomed to limbo. Her sister, Diane, often quoted something that F. Scott Fitzgerald once said—that the mark of true intelligence is the ability to hold two opposing thoughts in mind and still retain the ability to function. I heard my mother say quite often that spring that it was only life and death that were on the line.

When she met with the family lawyer, my mother was dying. She adjusted her will. When she attended meetings of the doctoral committee at Columbia, my mother was living, committing to events four months from the day. Her colleagues at the meetings, all social workers, delicately helped her manage at the meetings, taking notes for her, making sure that she felt up to speed, even if she could not be completely. It was important to them and to her that she remain a part of things.

She often said she had never been happier. She often said she felt at peace with everyone in her life. We had all grown comfortable in the waiting room between life and death. Grown comfortable in our discomfort. This was us. This disease was who we were. This is where we were, in June.

When I look back I can see that in many ways that spring and summer were a charmed time. She was losing more brain function than body function then. In fact, she was acing all her neurological exams. That woman could line one foot in front of the other for half the length of any hospital hallway. When she touched her nose with her eyes shut, NIH was like an audience at the Apollo—in love with a new act. We threw roses at her like it was opening night at the Met. She had become a show dog and the new her seemed to be satisfied with that.

She seemed calmer as she lost more cognitive ability. We could distract her, and she could distract herself with food and wheelchair rides, and for the first time, she saw a lot of "interesting things" on television. She especially got into Animal Planet. It was amusing to watch her engrossed in a dog's journey through physical rehab. *I'm rooting for the golden-poo,* she said, *big car accident. Barely survived. I can relate.*

It sounds diminutive, but she was cute during this time—like a mischievous elf. Just when you had written her off as a lobotomy case, she would come out with a clever quip to knock you one. She was always charming.

You'd say something inane like, *I just saw Jon Stewart on TV.*

And she would say, *Well, the next time you see Stewart, tell him he can go fuck himself.* It wasn't a particularly funny joke, but it was funny the way she said it. She was a grouchy little gremlin who harrumphed and cackled at the sound of swear words when she said them.

The mischievous smile would creep on at odd moments. She got her kicks in the summer. Anything went. She had us all rolling in the aisles. Her eyes had become so matter-of-fact. They tended to stare; they tended to stay where they had started. When she turned them toward you, it meant more than it once had. It was punctuation—an underline. Her eyes, once so animated, were like anchors now. She was free-floating and then she'd sink her eyes into you—and say something dry and amusing.

In that summer, sometimes I felt like she was our baby. We doted upon her. My aunt and I wrote down everything she said. We watched her watch television and giggled at her sweet, sincere reactions. *Gimme a New York vitamin,* she'd say, gesturing with the good hand as we'd haul out from the closet the box of a hundred Godiva chocolates. Each week we'd replenish the stash with the feeling of normalcy one has while filling a gas tank. She still closed her eyes to eat chocolate. She would breathe through her nose until it was gone. We jumped over one another rushing to bring our new baby whatever she wanted. We took breaks because we trusted Myrna. It was a wonderful time while it lasted.

∽

Wake up!
  Wake up!
  In an empty house no one can hear us. It is the end of August, the night before I begin graduate school. I call my father on the cell phone. I feel like I can hear the blame in his voice. He is trapped, in a taxi, forty minutes away.
  When she hit the floor, my mother shook the books right from their shelves. They scattered all around her like rain. Then white foam came running from her mouth, mixing with blood on the floor. She gave a long, low groan and was silent. I thought for sure that she was dead, and I was shaking her. I was screaming into her like she was hollow and deep—a well that I was leaning into, throwing my voice down into the dark water. I flashed forward to a life of having this as my final memory of us. After all our ritual bedtime stories this would be the last one. This would bury all the others.
  Mama!
  Mommy!
  Only echoes in an empty house . . . No one can help us. We will die here. The dog is running, howling. I call 911, and the dispatcher asks me a thousand questions, but all I can answer is, *Hurry.* I crawl to her, dragging the phone along the floor. I'm shaking her hand. There is no noise but the dog and me. Then suddenly her eyes are fluttering, and she begins to stir. I tell her not to move. They close again.

Don't sleep! I am slapping her hands, her face. *What is your name? What is your name?* And she doesn't know. *Who am I? Who am I?* I shout. *You are my child.*

And then the paramedics arrive. There are questions. They are loading her onto the stretcher. She doesn't remember she has cancer. She finds out when they ask me her medical history. *Alex, you must be confused. I've never had cancer.*

I have to warn my children when I have them that a mother always breaks your heart in the end. It is a natural law unless the child goes first. We must prepare ourselves to do this to our children. The promises we make are bunk. Life begets death. That is all. My mother kept me from this truth for as long as she could. She promised me once that she wouldn't die until I was ready. She truly believed that. We had spent the day together. Hurricane Katrina was about to descend on New Orleans. We watched the news coverage all day, and we knew it was going to be bad. We watched the long lines of cars as people tried to flee their city.

I'm probably going to have to go out there with the Red Cross, she said.

Everything was fine when my father phoned to say that he was heading home. We asked him to bring us caramel ice cream. I had been drifting in and out of sleep when she got up. For a while she had been able to walk on her own to the bathroom. She had gained so much strength from her physical therapy.

She stood at the foot of the bed. The hurricane coverage droned on in the background. The dog had just peed on the floor, and she almost stepped in it. Stepping back she lost her balance. I watched her try to right herself, and I didn't move, thinking that she would. And so I was still sitting there staring from the bed when I saw her stiffen in the air and fall down in a perfectly rigid line.

She slammed against the floor so hard that it seemed impossible she could survive. And all the books she had read and stacked away, one against the other came tumbling down around her. That spot of blood has stained the wood.

The St. Luke's emergency room where she was taken was next to the Columbia campus where I would be attending school the next day. When I left her, I simply walked a handful of blocks and began my orientation at the school of social work.

I do not recall how long before she left the hospital that time, maybe twenty-four hours, maybe more while they made sure she was stable. Her face was bruised, but amazingly nothing had broken. She was in good spirits, apologetic for having frightened me, bemused, it seemed, by the concern across my face.

For my field placement I was assigned a position in the inpatient psychiatric ward at St. Barnabas Hospital in the Bronx. The floor that held the ward was called Kane 3, which I loved because it sounded ominous. For some reason the word "Kane" reminded me of torture. At that time I was drawn to anything that made me feel dark. I needed decoy situations through which I could grapple with the overwhelming fear that I now lived with every day. It did not occur to me that this motivation alone meant I was in no shape to function as a social worker. I acted normal when I met my supervisor. I appeared concerned. I appeared caring. I almost believed my own performance. If I could act normal, maybe I was fine. I had so little insight at that point. I was surviving by trying to flee my true emotional state. At first glance, the hospital was more rundown than what I was used to at Mount Sinai. Kane 3 was spare and dark and overlooked gray buildings. Off in the distance from one window, I could see government-issue housing that some of the patients called home.

I loved the darkness of the place. The patients roamed and paced and sang their way through the hallways. I met a man who insisted he was in the direct lineage of Jesus Christ, and every morning he would bless me. There was a woman who was slowly scratching through her skin, a little deeper, a little more tissue every time I saw her. On my first day there I was given two directions: never go into a patient's room, not even a woman's room, and never walk to the end of the hallway alone. This was to avoid attack, sexual or violent, from certain patients.

Along the hallway the bedrooms lined up like paintings of a thousand worlds, a thousand wars laid out in thick brush strokes. I couldn't know more than what these people had the energy, willingness, or ability to tell me.

Some of them suffered from mental illness. They would say, *I see him in my contact lens. He comes to me. I can't put it in, 'cause I'd rather not see.* The hallway ended abruptly at a giant window opening out onto the Bronx, where all the buildings and trees stretched out like the cells of a body. And through dirty windows the patients would stand and point to their distant homes.

My daughter is seven, one said, *where is she?*

My mother was wondering the same. She would call me from beyond that skyline I looked at and say, *Alex, where are you? Come home. Alex, is that really you?*

The television in Kane 3 had plastic casing. A line of tape stretched across the floor before the exit door. I was not allowed to unlock the door to leave unless all the patients were behind the line. Mine was a skeleton key that I used to open and close all the doors. I traveled between rooms, lighting them, leaving them in darkness, carrying records of stories my patients told me with ticks of Tourette's, roving eyes, fidgeting fingers, and always, it seemed, patience. They had so much patience with me. I heard stories of being raped and of raping others, told bold-faced, tearless, cloudy-eyed, and I, the little social worker in training asking that they repeat so I could get it all down. When I heard their stories, I weighed them against mine. I had to buck up, I told myself. I was so privileged. I was so spoiled. People die. My mother was dying. So what? I told myself. Look at these people's lives. My pain is nothing compared with theirs. I sat with a Rubik's Cube of emotions trying to line things up, and it did not make sense. And it made me feel anguished.

Then there were the women, broken-down but not crazy, needing to get back to their sons and daughters. Too annoyed to plead, too experienced to respect me, they would click their gum and check their nails as we spoke. The floor smelled like the lunch that day, like vegetables waiting in lukewarm liquid. My office was just a closet overlooking a caged alley in which a pigeon lay rotting. I watched it decompose until someone finally swept it away. I don't know why after all that time they did not just let it be. I was like that, fallen. I was stopped. I was lying here. And my mother would not come for me. Not ever again.

My supervisor had left for the day. She had given me a list of things to do. I looked down at it, assorted black slashes that I could not seem to read. I locked the door, as was the policy. The room felt small—the two barred windows. The dirty white walls. Suddenly I knew the room was wrong. This was my life and there was no way out.

I made a shallow cut along my wrist with scissors from my desk, disbelieving even as I did it that I was cutting my own flesh. My mother had always told me I would have to impress my father to get his full attention. I found my hand was dialing his number, my voice telling him what I had done. And he was already in a cab as he asked me repeatedly what I was doing with my hands. Should he call the police? I do not know why he believed me when I told him I would not cut any more. I think we both knew that all I really wanted was him back.

His face appeared through my office-door window. He was with the guard and my supervisor. He looked at me with new eyes as if he had missed something. I took my father's hand.

Beginning on that day we were careful, like new friends. My anger and mistrust faded away. It seemed to make him cry now, just holding hands, walking to the corner to get out of the house and to get dinner. He would cry when he sat next to my mother and she would comfort him. She looked confused as if the strange melancholic ways of us mortals were something she could pity but never understand. *There, there*, she would say with her voice distant, *now there, there.*

Sometimes I would catch a shade of something in her face. I wondered if it was a moment of sadness that came and went too fast for me to share in it with her. Or was it only a sort of resin, a dust blown from the surface of some nonverbal place inside, a last vestige of who she had been.

Sometimes I would creep around, spy—sneak up to try to catch the real thing. I never did. My mother would turn slowly and give a little smile. I'd put my arms around her, but I couldn't touch her. More and more I focused on my father. I noticed he was frail. I helped him over curbs, always ready to catch him in my arms. I imagined death was turning toward him. I watched the lines deepen in his face. And for the first time I thought, let death take my mother as long as it lets me keep him.

I watched the papers grow in my room. I felt the work pile up. I lost myself in a sea of graduate-school reading. I would wave to my mother from there. Our time lay in pockets of twenty minutes, promises of tea or napping, always later, when I found time for a break.

I took to making drawings for her during my time in Kane 3. I drew a cartoon with our dog, Emily, as the protagonist. She would sneak around the house spying on my mother so she could tell me all about it when I came home. My mother thought these were hilarious but never understood them. She liked the lines, she said. The lines were funny.

My mother no longer had the ability to follow drawings such as these, or any story for that matter. She could follow only those that came to her, those stories that she spoke. She had stopped taking in new information. It was as if she'd left the island where we all were, on a solitary boat, pushed off the coast. She could tell us what she saw in the crystal blue water, or when it was murky, but she knew nothing of our island anymore. She knew only what she had already lived, that which she stirred in her crystal blue water. She rode her mind as it wandered, understanding things if and only if they were coming from her. Recycling old thoughts was easier than making new ones.

I could no longer see the surface of my desk. I watched the work pile up, cluttering, turning the desk into an old beached ship I crawled into and out from, grabbing artifacts to shove into shoulder bags—things I supposedly was working on, but in truth only picking up and putting down.

Each day I would rise to see that rotting ship. I could no longer find the surface beneath the mess, and I would just pass right by. I began to arrive late at St. Barnabas. I could barely stay awake when I was there. I devoured coffee and M&M's in the courtyards at lunch, cooped up in a narrow slit of sunlight. At the end of October I dropped out of school.

One day she could no longer walk at all. She had lost so much strength since her fall. One night I stayed sitting by her bed longer than usual because she seemed different. She was moving her mouth as if she were talking, but she made no sound. She gestured with her hands.

I stayed all night watching as she looked out into the bedroom, making welcoming gestures as if she were receiving much-awaited guests. The next morning I asked her who had been there. *It was my father in a death car*, she told me.

I had read that it was common for the dying to have visions of the dead. I called her two big brothers and her sister and told them they should come. Within a day they were all at our house. And as if on cue, she became lucid upon their arrival. She was lying in bed when her brothers walked in, and she perked right up. *Well, hello there*, she said. *I see the chickens have come home to roost.* It was a resurrection. It was as if instead of dying, she had decided to enjoy a good visit with her family.

It was the first time in years that the four siblings had been alone together. And they all said it was the best time they had ever had together. My mother was smiling the entire time that they were there. Those autumn days were sunny, and her sister and brothers rolled her around Central Park in her wheelchair. She was bundled up and fat, and she was happy. That was October. That was the last little good pocket of time we ever had.

Life happens in a rush in a hospital bed. It happens in the boxed-off squares of a calendar. It is perpetually closing in around us. There is no trapdoor to another way. When we commit to love, we commit to seeing death up close. In November, death was everything.

I think the steroids held her back too long. The fall colors muted in the frost. My father, Diane, and I had fielded family calls throughout her illness. We were so careful when we visited Minnesota, never leaving her alone with anyone we didn't trust.

When I phoned her siblings in October to tell them I thought she was close to death, her niece Donna responded too and came in a panic, without really asking. I was frustrated, but I also understood. My mother was her favorite aunt and her godmother.

On her first day in New York, we spoke more than we had in my entire life. Her stories showed me that she understood who my mother really was. By this point, everyone in our house was exhausted. My father and I were beyond tears.

Myrna Pedraza was spending five nights a week with Mom, so we had sent her home on a paid vacation. The conversations that we shared, the love she had expressed were in my mind when my cousin offered to spend the night in my mother's room.

I woke in the morning to my mother's niece whispering good-bye. And by the time that I knew anything, the niece was gone, flying back to Minnesota. I remember sitting on the bed and noticing that my mother couldn't move at all. It sounds crazy, but I was unsure of when it had happened. I wondered how long she had been like this.

I asked her to put her arms around me, but she could not manage them. The left hand hung limply on the wrist. The fingers wouldn't budge. So she brushed the back of her hand along my face. I remember thinking in that moment that her body was ruined and would never be repaired. The real her, in some ways, was becoming more visible now as if she were being peeled down to her true self, and that self had been ravaged.

I saw in her eyes all the things she longed to do, how much she longed to put her arms around me. No longer could she comfort with her touch. Her touch was just a reminder. She had become illness embodied. She had been turned into her own death. There was this big black cloud of smoke rising up around her. To be at her side had felt unbearable, like being locked inside a death chamber. To look upon her was to grieve. The strange child born of her disease that we had come to love was gone and this woman washed up, terribly changed, heartbreakingly familiar. She was broken in her body and her spirit.

She told me about the night before. She heard her niece crying. She felt her dead arm being pulled. Her niece was begging that she accept Jesus before she died. So in the end, despite all our efforts, they did come for her, came to claim what had so long been theirs. She had never really gotten out of that town.

I wonder if her niece ever felt a pang of guilt. I know my mom would have forgiven her. She would have said that we should speak no more about it.

We had a list of symptoms for nearing death. We had had it for a while—my aunt, my sisters, and I—at least through summer. And even in summer, we had been able to tick a few things off the list. We had it because we were all trying to be there when she died, and so we were focused on predicting when it would happen. We were always trying to figure out where she was along the timeline, what her status was, so we could prepare ourselves.

The list began at three to six weeks before death. The next category was two to three weeks before death, the next was one to two weeks before death, the next five to seven days before death, the next two to five days before death, the next eight to forty-eight hours before, the next was labeled "just hours," then "time of death," and then "shortly afterward."

I was worried about "loss of ability to swallow." I was afraid something terrible could happen, something violent that would take her painfully away. I made sure either my father or I was with her every time she ate. I read about CPR online.

I remember focusing on the "shortly afterward" section of the timeline. It read, "Many have commented that the face looks younger after death, the forehead looks free from wrinkles and cares, and the steroid bloating begins to disappear."

I yearned for her death for many months. Her disease allowed, or rather demanded from me, several states of mind. I could mourn her before she died while wishing her dead because of emotional exhaustion.

It was as if I were feeling sadness across time, both in the present and the future—like I was being tossed between two points.

My sisters were coming every weekend to help us, and my aunt Diane had come to stay indefinitely, which meant for the remainder of my mother's life. The air in the house was charged. I was morbid, euphoric, completely drawn out beyond all my reserves. I would tick off her symptoms as they happened. The chart became wrinkled and worn and lined with pen marks and scratch marks. Is it strange for me to say that it was an exciting time? I don't know what I thought would happen— that something really great waited for us all after she died. But what was that thing that I was thinking—simply a ceasing of pain? I began to imagine a house—Georgia O'Keefe's in the New Mexico desert. An adobe hut sitting in the sun. I wanted this place with no pictures on the walls and surrounded by warm earth. I wanted the special desert silence. The sun burning clean through my skin.

I deliberated over some of the items on the chart. Was she "difficult to rouse from sleep," as the list read, or only regularly drowsy? Was her abdomen distended, or was that merely the fat she had acquired because of the steroids she was taking? Were her motor movements weaker? I was completely of two minds. I still wanted to save her, but I also wanted to reach the end of the list.

Many have commented that the face looks younger . . . I wanted to reach release. I wanted to reach peace. Peace was what I had always associated with her. It was all she had ever given me. So in my mind, unconsciously, I married death to her return, as if reaching the end of the list would remove this heavy, sick, sad patient from my life and deliver to me my long-lost, cherished mother.

I remember it was nearing eleven. I was sitting at the kitchen table with my father when my aunt came in and pulled a chair up under long, wet eyes. And she told us that my mother had woken up and told her that it felt as if a body bag were being slowly zipped around her face. She said that she was struggling to breathe.

For days she had been staring at the wall in front of her, and Myrna Pedraza had taken on a pleading tone with me, a noticeable change from her usual calm. *Your mother isn't happy*, she would say. At first it seemed like a strange observation, but it wasn't. Throughout her illness, she had been, aside from agonized, aside from terrified, aside from valiant—actually, truly happy.

During the last two weeks I had asked her over and over again to share with me what she was feeling, what she was thinking, but she kept responding, *I am fine.* She had been disengaging me, I realize now, protecting me from her descent into something deep and final.

I phoned the doctor from the street outside. I remember I ran out with no coat on, though it was freezing. The air felt so alive, and I was pacing back and forth, looking up at her window as if at any moment my mother would appear and tell me to stop, that she was okay. That this was all a joke that I could get mad at, that I looked crazy down there making my circles in winter.

Into the phone I howled that she could not do this any longer. We were no longer doing right by her. My mother was completely paralyzed. She had stopped smiling altogether. For sixteen months she had fought, and now her body had been reduced to ruins, and she lay trapped inside it. My mother's treatment was never a treatment. In truth there were only three justifications for it. One, she wanted to try whatever it took to survive, and two, with glioblastoma, as her doctor said, there are no home runs. You can only work your way from one base to another and hope something will come for you. Some breakthrough in science, some discovery that can sustain you a little longer before too much of your brain has been consumed by the tumor and your body irreversibly ravaged—your ability to move and maneuver your limbs, words, and thoughts lost in subtle increments until your personality has been slaughtered and your essence barely remains. And the third reason was that my mother was a lab rat, and she knew it. Throughout her entire life, she wanted to be a pioneer in everything she did. She wanted to do the same with this. Deep down I know she wanted to be the magic lab rat, the brain that held the key, the canvas on which a cure would finally be revealed. She actually thought it might be possible.

There was never any real hope for my mother. Ours had been one more of the million against all odds stories that sum up the world every day. Life and time grow out of the fallen valiant bodies. To be the fallen valiant is our destiny. Whether we cheat it once or twice or a million times, we will all be buried under time.

She said she had had enough. My father listened. We all listened. We stopped the drugs and let the swelling in her brain cover her over like a heavy sheet of snow. She slipped into silence, never again took food and water. She slid into a deep, dark coma, but as she faded away, she held our hands. Her sense of smell seemed to stay, her hearing also. She touched my skin and a tear rolled down her cheek.

We were giving her morphine for pain. My sister Chris sat by her bedside dripping it onto her tongue when her breathing seemed labored. Her color started changing, bright red to deep purple to translucent green. She seemed illuminated from inside. Blue veins rose to the surface, then green, then capillaries. She was blushing, then sallow, then she was flushed again.

I stayed away for a while, lying on the living room floor. I tried to remember when it was that she stopped talking about living. My mother, Diane, and my sisters stayed by her bedside, holding her fingers as they became more limp, and her nail beds changed from light to dark. Something kept me from going in there. I did anything but that for most of the day. My mother had taught me as a child to be comfortable with death. It wasn't fear that kept me away. I felt that sitting in that room brought me no closer to her. Our connection was already growing somewhere else.

They had said it could take a week or more for her to completely slip away, but it was a handful of days. I remember being frightened she would wake up and it would begin all over again. But she would never again open her eyes. The drugs that we had stopped slipped from her like ribbons, let her loose, let her begin to roll away.

It was evening when Myrna woke me and led me into the bedroom. She told me that my mother was going to die tonight. I crawled into her bed with her as I had every day, several times a day, for the past sixteen months. I kept looking at her hand, where I could see every vein. Hours passed, and I felt so cramped in her bed. I got up and lay down between my father and sister on the other bed to rest, but I couldn't rest.

Everyone was half asleep around the room, chairs pulled along the bed, bodies lying at her hands and feet. Five minutes after I had moved, I went back. I climbed into the hospital bed. I was wrapping my arms around her when she died. I didn't even see it. By the time I looked up at her face, she had already gone.

I watched her for a long time. Her mouth was in a perfect O. It looked as if at any moment she would speak. In the end her dying felt like a birth to me, her last months an infancy. I didn't know where she had disappeared to when her breathing stopped. The possibilities unfolded before me in a long dark ribbon—like a road I once saw in Missouri, night driving, and she my only light as we moved along. She sat in the death seat beside me just as she did now.

When will we get there? I asked her all my life. Soon, she would say. Just concentrate, be patient. Just as a mother knows not the fate of her newborn child, I was blind to my mother's future now that she had left us. Yet throughout her illness, I had the sense I was preparing her for something great, something bigger than us both. Every bath felt like a baptism. Every kiss was as sweet as our last. I lingered often—held on to her hands, lay in her bed with her every day of that fall. I tried to have faith in the universe. I prayed for the first time. Please protect this child.

Just as a baby learns to crawl, she learned to lie down. She learned to take stock of her life and each day to let a little more of it go, a little walking, a little being awake, a little joy. Fall would calm her. By October she was laughing less; in consequence, we were laughing less. Maybe the reason babies cannot talk is because of what they would tell us. Like the dead, they are silent about what they know, and so the secrets of the universe are kept. Despite what my mother's family says, I think that the truth of the universe eludes us still. It is up to us to define for ourselves and, like Candide to spend our time tending gardens with care.

The moment I woke I glanced at the clock. Before I could let myself feel, I checked the time to mark my new life. My mother was newborn into death. She had left seven hours ago.

There ought to be a name for those who grieve. Though our bodies are alive, we do not live. We are not among the living but stowaways, trying to blend in and so angry that we have to even try, wanting at once to just throw ourselves into that fire, that dark water, after the one who left us.

I had dreamed of her confined to thrashing in the sea and I confined to watch her from a ship tossed with no direction in wet black. In this dream I feel my legs will walk me over. I wake worried that I dream so much of jumping.

The morning after she left, Dad and I let drop the last of the armor we had donned during her illness. We walked from that cover out into a silent, drafty house. She had torn through it with her dying, windows open letting in the winter bite, curtains tied up into knots, piles of sheets, her hospital bed already folded. My mother was everywhere but gone.

Dad sat down in a chair as old men do. Dozed off in the chair as old men do who do not want to sleep in their own bed. He moved seamlessly in and out of consciousness, seemed to dream awake. And in the psychedelic setting sun I saw him join the birds over the park and commence to fly back, back over those months. I knew then what it had required—the absence of her—for him to understand what he had done.

Now she was there in the pupil of his eye, lady beyond reach, cradled in the circle of the moon. Now they were facing one another in a way that they had not since before my mother was sick. They were marrying again. I don't recall whether it was that first day, but I know it was not that much longer before he said aloud to the room in which we sat,

I have failed you.

In the days that followed, Diane and I fought for the first time. There was someone she didn't want to speak at the memorial. She said he would not do my mother right. But I wanted no more of her or my mother's editing. If he was going up there to say all the wrong things, then I wanted to hear them. My mother was gone. And so should be her obsessive curation of us all.

Desperate to unleash my rage at Diane—for daring to express a need when it was my loss that I felt was the largest—I began to walk the house. I wanted to rip up the wood boards with my toenails, scrape my feet along the filthy underneath, picking all up, tearing the skin on the bottom of my feet. I would tear my face and spit my blood on her. Through the dining room I went into the kitchen, through the kitchen out into the hall, toward the windows of the living room, where my mother had sat so many days at that damn desk, a prisoner inside herself. I walked back to the hall again. I found a vase in my hand, heavy and crystal. I smashed it to the floor. Diane stayed silent in the next room, packing her belongings in a suitcase. Cindy grabbed my hand and took me out to walk me.

The memorial was just as my mother would have wanted. Piazzolla played from the speakers out over the church. There were so many people; there were hundreds. She never would have believed how many came. It was strange to see them all at once. I wanted to celebrate, to gather them all into my arms. I was visiting years of my life all in one moment, disparate eras, different countries where we'd lived; different ages I had been. There were so many travelers from far away.

There were times when she was sick she felt the world had forgotten her, abandoned her already. But it seemed today that the world had been loyal—as loyal as it can be for as busy as it is.

The world had come by her bedside, but all its words had lost their meaning. That was what she said. That was how she often felt. The world would come and pat her like a pet. She didn't want her new position at the center of a bed, hostess to the horrified, furrowed brow and well-planned praise, insistence that they meet again to talk—most people played the role of visitor that way.

In truth there was nothing anybody could have said that would have made her feel that she was not alone. Now, they were all here.

I felt triumphant—like she and I and our small family had been working, slaving away on something in secret, and now it was the moment to finally share. We had proof of suffering here. All those months in our apartment, we had been working on our little Frankenstein. We had produced our corpse, and all that we needed to complete this was their tears.

My mother's brother Donald was upset that she had not died identifying as a Christian in the way he understood it. In the light refracted into rainbows through the stained glass among the warm bodies of hundreds who had loved her, his conclusion was, *All her good deeds add up to nothing in the eyes of God.*

I heard my mother tell me to keep my head down and be gracious.

Gracious?

How her rules had enraged me growing up, though I didn't understand why they felt wrong. I idolized her, so I could not untangle my anger from my love.

So on the day that we remembered her, I shut my mouth in honor of my mother's Minnesota. I felt as hollow as a wooden doll that my mother made speak or be silent. Donald's words frightened me, because I shared his fear of hell. The idea of hell had terrified her, and though she never could say those words to me, she had transmitted that fear to me. Growing up, I was equally influenced by agnosticism and fundamentalism.

Diane was enraged when she heard Donald's comment. She had worked so hard to protect her sister all those months from exactly that, but the hateful words of their family had broken through.

She wrote to me, *I feel that I have lost them because of the choices they have made. The veil drops on the illusion that they cared about who I was. I am now the matriarch of my family. I'm not a sister or a daughter anymore. I'm a matriarch. An elder.*

I read those words not knowing what they would come to mean to me. Someday they would turn me like a wind dial, set me on a course I would not know I was on for a long time.

Just after the memorial, some friends took me to Florida. We stayed at a friend's father's house in Palm Beach. We drove to Miami in his car and stayed at the Ritz. We stole everything that wasn't nailed down, which was really just bathrobes and bathroom slippers. We were smoking then. We were drinking. We pranced around, forming a parade toward forgetting. We turned circles at night, getting more and more drunk underneath moon and palm tree, running along the water's edge, laughing until morning.

I was keenly aware of a certain phone call that I did not worry about making. I felt free but abandoned, and then a strange certainty that this separation was not final. We would meet again and again. But maybe that is just the kind of thought that occurs to you underneath the moonlight. It didn't last. My friends and I went back to New York and back to winter.

Before my mother was sick, I would become frightened sometimes when I was alone in my parents' house. Now I am captivated by every strange sound. Sadness makes me want solitude. Loneliness makes me want to hear a certain noise somewhere inside my mother's house.

I was walking the black length of my bedroom at night, well past the hour of phone calls and contact. I felt that if a hand were to come out of the dark, I would not shrink when it touched me. I expected the hand and I was waiting—walking toward it.

I filled my days with what I deemed normal behavior—mainly so I would not forget what it was. I had taken a retail job at a clothing designer's store managed by a friend. I sat on a high wooden stool, draped in the designer's clothes, breathing in and out the seventy-five-dollar scented candle, saying hello. Good-bye. Hello. Good-bye, as people came walking in and out. I would go to the back to check for sizes or to eat my lunch in little intervals. I drank a lot of water. I would bring two 1.5 liter bottles in the morning and finish them by the end of the day. I felt certain that if I did not eat, or drink enough water I would fall apart. I walked around the shop, straightening the clothing on the racks. I fretted over the credit card machine that I was certain would one day leave me in the lurch in front of a client. Even though I had learned to use the thing,

I never expected it to work. I don't recall that it failed me once, but I had no trust in it.

I watched the girls around my age come in and go out, sometimes I even knew them, sort of knew them. We would chat, I a little embarrassed, imagining them walking off to their important careers, and here I was working with girls six years younger than I, worrying I could not tame the credit card machine.

I don't know how you're functioning, the store's manager said. She seemed to do everything with ease. She seemed to do everything with confidence. I felt she could see through me. Had she not given me this job out of pity because our mutual friend had described the shape my life had taken? I imagined she could see my nerves, my sense of nonbelonging. The terror that crouched just behind my casual conversations with the clients, the effort it took for me to punctuate my personality with the occasional joke. Everything was such tremendous work.

When things were slow in the shop, I would begin to dream. Now the dead seem like an elite club. They sit like a parliament in my mind. I consult them. I have filled the chairs of their grand hall with all the people of my childhood. At this point the idea of ghosts are a comfort, would be a sign that my dark cottage has a back door, that pain is a process, not a destination where I have come to live out the rest of my days.

Not friends, not family, not books, not some last-minute fox hole jerry-rigged religion could care for me now. I need a ghost. I need a meeting place—a time off from the limited minds of the living. When my mother went, blood and feeling crossed with her, and it was life that seemed a gamble. It was death that stood with his feet on the ground. It was life that I could not be sure of. Death was real but life yet to be proven.

As Christmas drew close, Dad and I decided we should leave. We planned a trip to see my niece Corinne in Mexico. She was living in Puebla, working as an English teacher.

I sat in the plane staring down at what I had written. *Only your father can make himself happy.* I could almost hear my mother say it. But I had to make him happy.

The plane began to rock, the passengers stirred in alarm. I could not catch my breath. I looked back for the flight attendants to see if they were scared—they were doubled over laughing about something. Dad never looked up from his book. Did he not care either way?

I had flown into this city once before when I was a child but had refused to look. I had buried my face in my mother's arm as she described what she could see out her window. She was right. We fly so low over the city I feel as if we will land on a rooftop.

Christmas Eve dinner we had mole in a candlelit restaurant. Dad smiled when he spoke but not when he was silent. He would rest his cheek against his palm and draw with his fork along the tablecloth, lines that disappeared.

Without my mother we arrived everywhere on time or with time to spare. This was Bob with no Myrna around to make him late. Finally he could arrive early, and it was joyless. It was empty.

Travel with Mom was getting lost, marathon conversations, in hotels, in motels, and in other people's homes. In strange lands her mind wandered. She would take me walking as if the place had always been ours. We stumbled onto things. We never planned. And that is why it felt as if we ourselves uncovered museums, discovered monuments into being. Dad would be on his own spree, sleeping light and quick, waking early, running to anyplace that had any importance. Come seven o'clock he would be waiting in the lobby or in a garden or out on a veranda. His hair would be combed wet from a two-minute shower. He would be reading the *Herald Tribune* or a novel by a local writer or a guidebook as if it were a novel.

We laughed. They let me in on every joke. We talked about every thing, our life at home as seen from this new place. She would rib him over his being a nerd, about standing at the front of the line next to the tour guide, Berlitz under one arm, his double-jointed legs making him appear quite like a boy still growing awkwardly into himself.

In Mexico he still looked like a boy even at seventy-seven. His thick white hair fell over his face youthfully, almost demanding to be tousled.

We walked arm in arm, sat close to one another. There was an aura of protection as if we each believed the other was more fragile.

Traveling like this made me think of Minnesota country roads way out past town, where she and I would walk telling each other secrets. In Mexico it occurred to me that in some way she and I grew up together. She was thirteen, fourteen with me revisiting a time in which she wished she could have been happy. I told her everything, knowing that she would find a way to understand. And she was often thrilled by the same rebellions that were so thrilling to me.

We were always shutting doors on quiet rooms to whisper, one of us leaning on the door, the other fanning words like smoke, a reminder to speak softly. She endlessly observed every person she met. She picked people apart, not cruelly but with concentration as if she were pinning their bodies to wax paper to understand a species not her own.

To her I could say anything. And I could unsay it. And it would disappear. There was no crack in us, no black hole to fall through. Our relationship was safe. So safe we could think out loud together. We knew how to forgive and we naturally forgot. After she was sick that was no longer true and some things I said, some mistakes I made were permanent. They were the sword through us slain on the battleground. I did not let her stop at the Grand Canyon that time we drove cross-country, I was in such a hurry. And one day when she was yelling at me for having lost her wallet—when I knew she had lost it; she lost it everyday—I muttered that she was a piece of shit. A *piece of shit?* What had I even meant? It made no sense. Who says that to their mother?

I cry in the hotel bed trying not to wake Corinne. I watch the shadows move across the ceiling as cars pass by outside. I remember shadows and her voice in hotels and motels, and other people's homes, the sound of her speaking in the darkness, the indescribable feeling of being another woman's child.

I am not sure Dad and I saw Mexico. We treated that country like a faceless one-night stand. No regard for who it was just what we made it be. We were dreaming. The world was her toy, a dollhouse in which she moved all things. Everything that happened she made happen, all of it was intended for us.

I felt her, Dad told me, *as I waited for you, felt a hand on my shoulder and I turned expecting . . .*

I love you, I said to the stray dog that stopped beneath the moonlight to console me.

✑

I cannot see myself. I do not know how to live my life. And I hate it when people ask me how I am. And I hate it when people do not. Days are not mine to know how to fill. I yell at myself that I am not doing better. I wonder whether misery is a choice or whether it is the other way around and misery chose me. And then I am angry with myself for being helpless.

I dreamed that the world was the size of a tennis ball beneath my feet, and I was running madly to stay on, left foot, right foot, left foot, right foot—one single mistake, and I would be falling through firmament, grasping for the blackness and the stars.

I think about things. I remember how the cold air was trapped in my mother's coat when she came home at night, and she smelled like the street and like winter. I remember I would greet her at the front door in my Bert-and-Ernie slippers. But as the years passed I didn't always greet her at the door. I thought we had time. I thought I had more years to show her how happy it made me each time that she came home.

I remember the night of her seizure when I had thought that she would die, and the Haitian woman, how nobody spoke Creole and every few days, if she was lucky, they would call in that French doctor.

They had made a chart for her room. It read, Bathroom. Pain. Nauseous. Help me. Hungry. Next to each item there was a circle drawing of a face with a different expression. This woman had bone cancer. She is definitely dead now too.

I remember how much Mom and I hated the male nurse on our ward. I lay in bed with her, and we whispered about him. We whispered that if killing by hospital staff were legal, he would do it. I wondered what this man could have against my mom—this sweet, doped-up woman who tried to smile every time he came in. We decided to refuse his medication. We were going to demand another nurse. We needed protection. But his shift ended too soon for us to do this, and we were relieved. He was the night nurse, typecast for the graveyard shift. In the first rays of the morning light, he vanished.

We whispered about all the people in New York right at that moment who were sick and at the whim of someone like him. We thought about the people who were more alone than we were and more helpless. It seemed that a giant part of being sick was being beat on in a way. Doctors were hurried, distracted, and vain, nurses and nurse's aides were overworked, underpaid, and so many seemed angry.

I saw so much wrong in the hospital. All night voices would cry out from their rooms and find no answer. I would wander to their door, walk by to look in, and see one curled up like a raven's claw halfway off its bed, broken and forgotten. They whispered, *Help me. Please, help me.*

This is how so many of us will end our lives. Although most of us never think of it, the hospitals are filled with us, already forgotten.

I fold over memories, smooth them, run my hands along them, go feeling for her. I think of when I was small enough to climb up onto the kitchen counter and have my hair washed up in the sink, how much I loved that feeling. I would stare at the ceiling lights until I had to close my eyes. Then I would watch the colored circles run against the black. I would lie on my back, my finger fiddling with the kettle button.

When my body is zipped up in the black bag, I want to remember that warm kitchen and my mother's fingers moving through my hair. I must be dreaming. I wake up, and the day has left me. The room is doing an impersonation of my head—disorder reigns. When did she die, how long ago?

This is winter. Today is the last day of January, and I know the worst is yet to come. In February, the cold will no longer feel new. Then March that always disappoints, that endlessly surprises me with all its cold indifference. Then April the flowers she loved but will not see. I wake up. I pass the winter dreaming in this way.

That winter I touched the bottom of something. I gave up on trying to make things better, stopped dead in my tracks. It didn't seem that I could ever find my life. The house stayed dark. The dishes grew out of the sink—higher and higher, ready to tip over the edge of the counter. In the months after my mother, I could not control my anger. It was directed at everyone at any time. I watched the words roll out from me—a horrified spectator, able only to watch the carpet roll and wait to see what would come parading down it.

I was lonely. Life was ending, always ending, and too slowly. January, lonely January has been a strange time—nights and dreams and productive busy solitude, though productive of what I am not sure. There are dinners with friends, agreements to quit smoking, and books, books, books.

I spoke often with my sisters on the phone. They had become my only real friends. They were the only people I felt I could trust to be myself with. With everyone else I wore a brave face, not creepy with unfeeling but a face nevertheless false. If people had known the depth of my need, they would have been horrified.

February, cry though you feel nothing. There is only the physical feeling; a grip around your neck, your insides scraped clean by some kind of demon's fork. I walk to her bench on Eighty-sixth where we used to sit. I try to weep but only sit. I force myself to wait in the bitter cold until the tears give up and come. It feels strange to cry out in New York. I realize how rarely I see other people do it, even though in this city you live on top of one another. I don't know how it is that I observe so little. Maybe something makes me look away. Maybe that is a human talent.

I move on from the bench—walking, hiding my hands in my coat. I haunt the city, and the city haunts me. I know no one anymore. I stay in my head now. Ideas go by all day. The subway cars are packed with them. There are messages in everything, stories that the other riders tell me while I pretend that I'm not listening. I probably communicate things too. No one knows what we mean to one another when we are not talking, when we're strangers.

My mother speaks to me through a gathering of strangers, says to me everything she can no longer say. I see the world dance along with the swing of her baton. How will I ever get over her if I cannot get away? She is everywhere the mind can hide. She is in every book and every letter, every word. She is woven into the tiny grains of paper.

Sometimes I catch a glance, and I think it knows me, and I know it too. But then it darts away; the glance is again a stranger's face. There is a moment before words make themselves necessary. There is a truth in the stare before a smile. You find sadness like this, painted broadly over faces, and then as if by order, heads will turn.

A letter arrived today that smelled of the hospital. If you knew, you would say to these forces haunting me, *Leave my girl alone.* You would never have thought I would stop living to dream about you. This is what I do. I can still see you in your bed, lying paralyzed. You said life had revealed itself to you. You said, *I have never been happier.*

You used to say that all the time when you were sick, and you weren't faking. You really felt that way. That was the genius of you, ever the artist making beauty out of what others call fact. I used to worry about whether you were more yourself as you were living or as you were dying. I do not worry anymore. You were both.

Today I walked by your old Victrola. All at once it was as if you were standing before me. I saw you in the way the room leaned. In the picture frames and the books as you left them there on the piano. I thought of how someday my child would stand staring at my things—remembering how I had stacked them up and refusing to move one, in February.

God or Minnesota or whatever to call you, I know that I have not been religious. But you must understand I've lost someone. She and I came into cancer together. I dream she has emerged somewhere with you. I am still here. In the still that lies here, staring at the spot where she once was. I cannot see anything beyond this empty spot. I am asking for her back. I will give anything in return, in winter.

☙

In the first eleven years of my life when they would take me traveling so often for their work, my mother and I would swim out into lakes and seas to talk. We lost ourselves on foreign streets, in foreign cities, following our words for hours, losing our way a million times, asking again and never listening how to get back to our hotel.

By the time that we arrived, much later than we should have, Dad would be worried, his arms folded. My mother and I would tease him, throw our arms around him and soften him up.

Once, we got to talking in a zoo in Buenos Aires and it closed, locking us in. We walked around searching for an escape. The animals hollered and jumped and followed us as far as they could before they reached the ends of their cages. They were alarmed it seemed to see us in the near darkness out of the regular context.

We were jumpy and spooked and in hysterics, laughing so hard we doubled over. My mother said we'd have to climb the wall. My father happened to arrive as I threw my first leg over the top of the metal fence at the zoo's entrance. He was angry and worried and also, after taking in our mood, he felt excluded.

I feel left out, he always said. *You guys are leaving me out.*

A grieving mind plays tricks. It's petulant, won't let you do the work of life. You have to raise it. You have to grow it fat and wait until it is strong enough to want to leave you, find someone else to drink from like a mother.

The phone rings, and for a moment I expect it will be her. In February I have been spending far, far too much time alone. What I do is not called life. I wait in a heart that wants death. The heart lies with her now. I feel that I cannot have it back. It goes beating far away, distracting, calling me to it.

When night comes I cross countries running, as if on four legs, I move through trees and water, my muscles beating to the sound of a distant metronome that sat so many years ago atop my mother's piano. The vibration of its hum shakes the earth I walk on like a flimsy planet. I awake exhausted. My dreaming life is swallowing my days.

I feel left out. You are leaving me out.

I backed into the hallway in the morning, staring at the ancestors framed upon my wall. I should put her picture there for she has gone as far as they. I hear the click of the front door close behind me, feel the hand upon my shoulder. Turn. Turn. And face your father. The only one waiting is you. Only one coming home is he. Even in that ache something felt right. Something felt late as if it had been pending. I had had to lose my mother to truly know my dad.

We began to confide in each other in small bursts, then we would both recede, not to a place of alienation but of pacing. We wanted to protect one another. Neither of us could bear the thought of further loss. We were bound by grief, and that old friendship that formed during my childhood returned like an old dog showing no lack of loyalty despite our having banished it.

Dad became the old man that he was. I took his arm on winter streets. I held my palm to the crown of his head when he lowered his body into cabs. I loved him in a way that broke my heart every moment that I loved him. I was grateful that I had some time to love that way. We lived so very much in the moment. It was all we had any energy for. All that mattered was that right now we could be together.

I make many lists in March. The lists scream for much-needed attention. I go about my business on a Saturday morning, minute details of coffee—the machine leaks brown sludge and I wipe it off the counter every day. I'm pouring out the cereal, filling Emily's bowl, and I'll remember my mother's face hitting the floor. In all the blood, the day just dies, pulls itself up to the bar to order a drink before noon. I hit her La-Z-Boy, and the music of TV fills the air. What's another day.

Since my mother died, I break all my own promises. I have no motivation to be disciplined. I wake up sad, and I don't change my life. I work the same dumb job at the film studio. It does not feel like change is a choice. I don't remember why I ever did hard things. On a good day I keep motivation up till the third quarter. I stopped on the way to the post office today. I didn't feel as if I could go on. I didn't feel like turning back. I held on to a stoop for a long while as if it were the only thing I could find to cling to in a liquid world.

Last night I think we spoke. I awoke this morning and felt you had been here. I could almost make out your imprint on my chair. Last night did you tell me something? I have the feeling I was told a secret, but I cannot recall.

I join the cast of a play, a friend of a friend. The actress dropped out and they need someone last-minute. This is good, I think. It gives me a place outside of work I have to be at a certain hour every day. It specifies a time in which I must appear to function as a normal person. This is good, I think. It is a time when I cannot act crazy. Acting crazy is talking to her picture, turning circles in her closet. Going through her things nervously as if at any moment she might walk in.

On the wall of her closet, there is a list she made of outfits, down to the belt. I stand inside and close the door, try and get her smell. I stick my face into her old fur coat. Her closet is the only place to find her arms and have them reach around me. Or sometimes I go in there not to be with her, but because I need to borrow something. I always put it back when I am done. Maybe it is a shirt that I need. During these times, there is a voice that I push down, a child's. I cannot listen to what it says as I search for a shirt. I'm going out into the world—that's right—and have nothing to wear to this play rehearsal.

The city bus has stayed the same. The buildings are standing. The moon has not rolled away. But everything for me is skewed. In my dreams, the world is a globe on my bed stand. I spin it once searching. She is nowhere to be found. I get on the bus to go to rehearsal. I leave early to ride the bus to search for her. The bus is slow in New York, except when it winds through the park, making me dizzy. I remember her standing too close to the edge of the curb, rustling through that oversized purse she always carried. Rehearsal is the only time that I forget her and lose myself in play.

I imagine correspondence. I think that she sends messages to me, or maybe I have memorized her, and I send them from her to myself over and over. Maybe it is as if I have continued writing lines for her dead character. I'm seeing everything in terms of dialogue now because of the play. The world around me has become a means of measuring comedic or dramatic timing, a vast buffet of words and ideas to steal from. I make notes wherever I go.

When I was young I used to build cities that stretched across whole rooms in my parents' house. They would come home from work and have to maneuver around them. They never made me take them down, because they valued them. They knew that for a child that was work. Alarm clocks were grandfather clocks, tissues were bedsheets, and coasters were expensive works of art on dollhouse walls.

Now a line of papers covers the floor of my father's front hallway. I keep shifting them around. My plan is to write about the whole thing. To make something of it.

In my childhood constructions there were cities and marriages and murders. There were towns whose serialized stories went on for years, starting and pausing with the coming and leaving of nieces and nephews and cousins. In these games, my dolls spoke to me as my mother does now. So I see that long before her, I was receiving messages. I see that a vast part of my life has been a dream world in which I was no less than confined. A great part of my life has been my imagined life. A story I am secretly telling myself. So many of my surroundings are of my past. My ladies-in-waiting are ghosts. If it weren't for the dead, I would spend most of my time alone in March.

There was a homeless woman on West Fourth Street at the subway stop. I smiled at her one day in winter. She made me think of that old show *Quantum Leap* that I used to watch with Grandma Easter. At the end of every episode, the protagonist is transported to a new time and place. He might find himself in a Nazi uniform, or a dress, and he's trying to learn his surroundings before anybody notices that he's strange.

This woman was acting as if she had touched down and still didn't know she was a homeless woman on West Fourth. She was looking down at her rags and her garbage bags and then out at the reactions of people, as if she was processing it all. Then she saw me watching her, and she gave a look of recognition as the doors started closing on the car. She said, *Daughter, be happy.*

Mother, I thought when you died the old you would come back. I wanted so much for the illness to end that I separated the death of you from it. I thought you would come back and say, *I've been watching you and you tried hard, Alex. And you did as well as you could.*

In the building where you used to live, from the elevator before the door closes, sometimes I'll see a car pull up on the street outside, and I will expect you. I will expect you so much that I will see you. I will see you through the dirty window of the cab. And you'll come running. You will practically fly out. You were always in a rush. You were often late. It used to make me mad, but now I'm counting on it. You have to be running late.

I used to walk into the park to get away from you when you were sick. Now I go there to imagine you are home, waiting for me. You have been replaced by the things you used to do. Now I do them. You used to walk in the Shakespeare Garden; now I do. You used to like Gray's Papaya; now I do. I see movies alone. I keep my coat in a second seat. I walk for hours. I listen to books on tape. I channel you. I imagine I am you.

When I imagine I am you, I think about Alex. I wonder how to be her mother. I wonder how her life will unfold. Will I know how to advise her? Will I do it well? I worry, sometimes, that I will run out of words to console myself with. That I will run out of memories to draw from. I yearn for you, a kind of pain that is so dull I cannot find it, that is so sharp I dumb it down. It hides from me, deep within, beyond all effort I can make to find it. When I think how I am helpless in this, when I wonder if I will have this pain all my life, I start to panic. But then it comes to me. I know what you would say, *Just keep walking; it is spring in Central Park.*

I have a letter from you. You wrote it when I was fifteen. You were traveling on a six-thousand-mile trip on a train from Helsinki to Beijing for the Beijing Women's Conference. The trip was considered somewhat dangerous, and so you decided to write me this letter—a list of twenty things, your most important beliefs about life. In the last months of your life you searched frantically for the letter, but you never found it. I found it.

Alex, my sweet and dear child, I expect to live to a very old age so I can see how you put your life together, and take pleasure in watching you do it. But if for some reason I die early, you carry on. (In spite of your dramatic declarations to the contrary at age fifteen. Do you remember?) Life is often inexplicable—but loving intensely and passionately is what makes all the sense in the world. Do a good job of this, my girl. Your loving mama.

I expected spring to bring so much, but it led nowhere. And summer was so slow to come, like water set to boil. It had me waiting. Then all at once I felt the heat and knew I had to jump if I was going to survive.

Somebody offered me a ledge. Someone I had known before her illness, when I had lived the life of a privileged youth who could chase trouble before it chased her back.

I lied to my father, saying I was visiting a friend up north, but I was headed south on a train, with my heart jumping. I had not seen him in so long, though we had spoken on and off during her illness.

He was not the same as I remembered. He said he had been suffering, that he had thought of my mom every day. He was thirty now, which seemed so old, and he looked kinder. And yet he still drove as I remembered, cursing every person he passed. I do not know why I felt safe in his car. That may have been what he did best, make me feel numb while he put me in danger.

We talked about everything that had gone wrong, and he said many things that I had wished for a long time he would say. He told me that despite their differences he had loved my mother and he had thought about her every day. It had broken his heart that she refused to take his call.

To imagine my mother horrified was too upsetting. I felt her push me forward, toward any kind of relief in any form. I pushed off into a new relationship with him. Because they had always been so separate, now that I was with him, I rarely thought of her.

I felt like a different person at his side. I barely recognized myself in his description of me. Yet I was young and dumb enough to think that he might, as goes the tired expression, know me better than I knew myself.

I did not say no, did not say yes. He told me to *grow up and figure out what it is you want.* Unfortunately, I thought I *was* old. Ever since I'd met him, he had offered to save me, and I had started to believe I needed it. Sometimes he would attack my background, my *haphazard upbringing.* He called me *the spoiled daughter of old, lenient parents.* He said that they had not really known me because they were old and out of touch. Sad that any daughter of my father would buy an ageist line like that.

Years later I would realize what drew me to him, what it was that rang a bell and made me follow him like a beast. His power over me reminded me of Mom.

My father did not try to stop me when I moved out. He said he wanted me to know I could always come home. He understood this was the only way I knew to move forward at that time.

It was raining. We stood beneath the building canopy. He held my hand through the taxi window. He stepped back from the taxi, and it pushed off into the inky street. The stoplight became red, I turned and looked back at him. He clutched the arms of his sweater tied over his shoulders. I could not believe that I could leave him. He looked so alone. He was seventy-eight years old. His beautiful white hair. But I had his dumb, deadly time bomb in my chest that I knew would blow up if I stayed. I had never been so certain that my life depended on one thing, and that thing was to run.

I was not strong, nor brave, nor possessed of dreams or any imagination. I wanted stillness and quiet, what this man had offered, to be carried; to be numbed and allowed to sleep.

A couple weeks after I moved in, it all dissolved. We had been fighting. We were on the stairs. I reached for him. He pushed me and I landed on a step, not too hurt, or even frightened, just perplexed, as if what was occurring were all a great mystery. As if I were an anthropologist trying to decode a strange and new behavior, not a woman getting pushed by a man onto a stair. His hand curled into a fist flush with my face. *You are a pathetic slut,* he said. *A zero.* I had confided in him that I had dated someone else. He had dated someone else. Apparently that was irrelevant.

I cocked my head to one side, allowing the sentence to bounce back and forth as if through the acoustics the reverberation of something underneath could become heard. I pitied him. Was this a man in pain? Was he confused? He seemed suddenly pathetic. A giggle made its way around my ribs as with a child on the monkey bars — I was conscious that I could not let it climb out of my throat. He turned and punched the wall with his fist.

That was not the first time that I did not cry when he said horrible things. Those words flew past me, held no claim. I felt shock and a strange nervous amusement at the arcane insults that he tossed like knives. They did not strike me as being much more than the ranting of a stupid hick out of a movie script, a song, out of a novel — a boy who lived in a low-down state, a low-down country, small town, small amount of teeth.

I did not believe in sluts. My mother had bought me condoms in eleventh grade. Sex was treated as a simple fact. I went to art schools, alternative high schools, Quaker camps where women counselors grew their body hair and shaved their heads, taught us songs about mythical women warriors, discussed gay rights, female objectification in the media. I understood these things at five and six.

He must be joking. He could not be serious. My high school boyfriend and I had shared each other's boxers, shaved each other's heads — worn each other's clothes. During one of our breakups, I dated a girl. He was completely unimpressed. He was jealous. He went out with her too.

I had grown so far from this kind of thinking that it felt exotic, and yet here I was on his stair, laid out like a rag—in fact a rag doll. I was my mother's rag doll left over from her abandoned life, cotton stuffing for my brain, my heart detachable, as easily stolen as if it had been sewn onto my chest.

He was ready to make up. He touched my arm for the first time gently. I felt that arm unattach from me. I floated off. He could do what he wanted. I would sleep that night next to a warm body. A warm body made sleep possible. To lie alone in bed was to lie with Mother.

I don't want a cane, she had said at the beginning, by the end such a small thing to have worried over when she would lose so much. But that cane was an affront to her pride and her identity. I had no pride. I had no identity. I slept like a dead woman in the house of a man whom I hated because it kept me from dreaming of her.

Every mother is made up of rituals, certain ones that maybe only her children can know. When I was growing up, my mother could make anywhere in the world feel like home. As a child this was important to me, traveling so often with my parents. I was always partial to routine. My mother had a purse that rivaled Mary Poppins's. It seemed to hold an endless array of toys and food, medicine in case I became ill, my full medical history.

Don't dig, Alexandra, she would say. Everything was in the same place, neatly organized inside her purse. I did not have to look to find my crayons and paper. They were always next to one of those mealy red apples so endemic to the 1980s.

She was sneaky, come to think of it. She would set up what she called play stations. One would be a pile of books, another a pile of blocks. She would find objects around the room and help me turn them into toys. When I became bored, she would come up with another game, or some kind of adventure. She would lean down from a conference table and whisper in my ear. There were many games of tic-tac-toe on table napkins that we would pass back and forth. I spent enough time under tables in my childhood to perfect the thrilling game of touching people's shoes without their knowing.

Wherever we were, she pointed out the simple lovely things, how each hotel made a slightly different grilled cheese, or how every city had *a special magic nook with our name on it* where she could read aloud *Rebecca, Jane Eyre, Wuthering Heights* as I acted out the stories with my dolls.

I drank a million Shirley Temples off room-service trays and watched black and white films on hotel TVs. Certain films have fused with certain places. *Annie* is from Beijing, *The Music Man* is Mexican, and *Casablanca* is a strange, anomalous town in the center of Vienna. Though travel so often felt like fever, like waking up in strange beds, having been transported in my sleep. Though daylight would arrive at the wrong time and bring with it a strange language splashing outside in the pool beyond my door, there would be her glasses folded on the nightstand, her book with the bookmark that her mother had sewn, her little container of Pond's Cold Cream.

And so I knew how to make myself feel at home anywhere, how to play alone, invent my own adventures. These things made me feel at home with this man. Yet in truth I was adrift, directionless, completely undeveloped, with no idea of what to do for work, living off this man and my dead mother's money that she had died too soon to spend. But I made a life in the way my mother taught me. It made me feel as if we were still together.

I began thinking often of how different I was from my parents. They were born with so much less than I. They had made their way themselves. I was an anomaly, I realized. My parents had made me feel I was like them. I was not like them. I was twenty-five now. My mother would have said, *The jig is up*. I felt that the person I had become was pathetic. I had mistaken my identity for theirs; because they loved me so, I had assumed that I had earned it. But now it occurred to me they would have loved any child born to them. My sense of uniqueness fell away in the absence of my mother. I grew as thin as tracing paper living with that man.

Every day I would wake up with a feeling of unease, every night a feeling of exhaustion. I called my father often and told him I felt fine. We spoke warmly, but he always said good-bye first. It seemed life had reabsorbed him. He was working all the time, he said. He had gone on a date with a woman.

I asked him how it was. I could almost hear him shrug. *Keep trying,* I said. I desperately wanted him to have someone—he seemed so alone. I had no complicated feelings about my father's finding love. I was in favor of anything that would keep him alive; that would keep him with me.

At least it is a night out, a nice conversation, a nice dinner, he said. *But nobody has your mother's mind. How are you?* he would ask, and I would say, *I'm really good. I'm really, really good.*

In 1998, on the day that I met the man for the first time, he held the zipper of his jacket in his teeth, up and down, up and down it went. He stared at me. He seemed different from anyone I had ever met. When we spoke, he would listen intently to everything I said. His eyes would narrow, his brow crinkle, he would nod. It is difficult to explain how well he did it. He was a real champ. I had this feeling right away that we understood each other, that we were connected; that we were already loved ones.

He was calmer than the other boys, more confident. He would shoot me a look when he left that made me want to drop onto the ground. He would wait for me, open the door when his friends forgot, not in a cheesy way, in an amazing way. But then all at once he would be distant, then back with me with this kind smile spreading across his face, and he would do a little something, not too much, nothing I could keep, a fleeting gesture like touching my cheek or squeezing my hand that seemed to signal he already loved me. This was us in the early days, few words, expansive, horrid silences and staring at each other with great meaning.

We fought more than we communicated, but then I would not let him leave, I would push him against the wall and bar the door. It was fever. I would follow him to where I knew he would be. He would tell me I was special and then disappear. All these things convinced me that there was no one else.

It is hard for me to identify with the girl who fell. It is hard to imagine yourself back into innocence. I wish I had fancied him a moment and then walked. I wish I had stopped him at that first conversation. Then all that man's pain and anguish that he gave me credit for could be called the evil work of another woman.

I didn't walk away, not even now. Though I thought of leaving every day. I kept filling my life with little things.

I became a teacher for small children who threw their arms around me every day and sang my name. I would stand in this cocoon of smiling children, each finger claimed by a different little hand, and try not to cry.

If I avoided certain subjects, the man and I would get along most of the time, sometimes surprisingly well. And yet I wasn't happy. And yet I did not have the energy to leave. And yet the world was shifting, not only my heart but my entire life as I had built it up after her death. And I started to think about the fact that it had been a year. I felt everything in and around me was coming down, hollow and false as a film set.

I thought of the boy I had met when my mom got sick. He had stayed with me through the rough first months, and he would have stayed longer, maybe—I don't know. One night as he and I were leaving to go out, Diane seemed to be drinking us in. *You are a young and handsome couple,* she said beaming. And then quite suddenly, inspiring in me equal parts horror and delight, she broke into a rendition of the classic show tune "Hello, Young Lovers" from *The King and I.* My mother's voice joined hers harmonizing from the bedroom. We backed out of the house and shut the door, leaning against it. We could still hear them from the elevator as it traveled down. *Call me a trouper,* he had said. I remembered distinctly what it felt like then to be with a nice person, the kind of confidence it could provide. I almost could not get in touch with that kind of comfort.

You need a psychiatrist! The man would scream, rattling the knob of the locked door to the bathroom. I began to imagine my mother coming for me. I imagined her swooping in to carry me out of there as she had often done throughout my life because I was too weak.

Years later when I would think back on that time, I would realize I had not so much been weak as flummoxed in my grief and fear, cut off completely from myself. It was as if I simply could not see that I could make my own way without someone who felt they knew better. I had superimposed the man where the mom had been.

Alex, you are starting to scare me. I think you need help. I understand that you believe that you are grieving, but it's been a year. But as someone who cares about you, I have to tell you, you don't see things as they truly are.

I read constantly, more than ever before in my life. I left and disappeared into the pages of books just as my mother had told me about doing in her childhood. I developed what felt like a telepathic connection with my dogs, complex and spiritual. They were my only comfort and I theirs.

Something was making me sick. I would wake an hour early before work so I could read and will myself to crawl out of my bed. To get up, bathe, walk the dogs, eat, bike to work took a feat of iron will. Work was a refuge. I would go to the classroom twenty minutes early to sit in total quiet, line the chalk up against the blackboard, check my face in the mirror to make sure I was real.

The students would arrive and I could lose myself in the flow of addressing their momentary needs. When the bell rang, I would awaken and watch them leave, relishing their friendly treatment of me. To them I was real. I could always act. At the end of the year, my student reviews were strong. I did not come home to the man. I went to a bar with the other teachers and became so drunk I wiped out three times riding my bike home.

I woke up still drunk and considered leaving, but I was terrified. He had never punched me, only slapped. He had never thrown me, just pushed and let me fall. Yet I believed he was capable of killing, maybe because in some way he was killing me each day.

I started to live as if I were undercover to trap him in an act, for which I could bring him down. I began to scrutinize him as if trying to make out electric gears that moved beneath his skin in place of blood. I took to reading about sociopaths. I decided that he was one. I organized all my belongings. I went through my school papers, threw most of them out, organized my closet, organized everything I had in a way so that it could be packed quickly. I knew just where everything was and which places held the most important items.

I looked at my reflection in the foggy window, high cheekbones and deep-set eyes just like my mother. We had the same mouth. And through the glass, from the mouth: *No one fucks with my girl. I will come like a mother lion.*

I started to hit him. I began to bait him to hit me. We would pinch each other under tables if one of us said something the other didn't like. We kicked each other too at crowded tables. Friends would shift uncomfortably in their seats. Our relationship started to feel eerie, as if we were both spies and both of us knew it.

Love you, I would say looking past him.

Love you.

You okay?

Just sad to see you go.

Me too.

Our faces did not go with our words.

It is possible to walk out of your life in a matter of days and leave all of it behind. In New York I told my friend everything. We were on a stoop fanning ourselves in the heat in hectic Soho complaining about Soho. She started to cry, which made me speak faster, buoyed by her reaction. These were the tears that I had lost, having floated so far from my heart. *I could come with you to move you out,* she said.

I told my father and my sisters everything as well. Now I had to leave, I thought, or I would slowly lose all these people. We would drift apart the way you do when everybody knows you've forsaken yourself. And just like that I left him.

When I was a child, I believed for a year that I was being followed. I would see the same face over and over in the crowd. I began to draw the face, realizing there were several, a group who disguised themselves with wigs and facial features made of clay. My father's mother, Easter, believed me. She tended to shoot from her right brain. We would try to lose them by getting on and off our bus at different stops each day. I would peer from the back window and watch the faces turn angrily.

That entire year I crawled past my bedroom window. There was construction down on the street below and I knew they were drilling secret patterns and codes all about me. I was not sure what these people wanted, but I understood that the safety of my family depended on me. My mission continued to obsess me until it faded some time at the start of the fifth grade.

Similarly I obsessed about the man, that he was coming for me, coming to hurt me. I realized one of the biggest gifts I had received from death was learning how to bury the living when need be. I changed my e-mail, my phone number, and I never heard from the man again. The string of e-mails that I had received before closing my account I would not let myself read. I had my sister check my e-mail for a while. I had her change the password so that I would not look and she saved anything from him that might contain a threat, then after a few weeks she closed the account. Years later I would look back on those e-mails with her, one from his sister, one from his brother, and one from an anonymous person berating me. That one read to me like Norman Bates. I envisioned the man dressed as someone else to write that e-mail, to pour all his hateful words out and at the same moment have the chance to describe himself in ideal terms as my victim. But by the time I read it, the spell had broken and I no longer fell for his lies. But all that was not, I think, the main point of what happened with the man. The main point was that I fought my first real battle without Mom.

So at twenty-seven I moved back in with my father. I felt like a loser, and yet I was so happy to be home. The house was heavy with his loneliness. I had been wrong to imagine that he was doing well. He had not called more because he wanted to let me live my life.

At night he would ask me to sit with him a minute when he got into bed. He still slept on his side of the bed. In general he took on the behavior of a house cat. I would be reading and turn to find he had curled up in a chair near to me and drifted to sleep.

Mornings he would patter out in his pajamas and robe. He would open the front door and bend down slowly, making sure to bend his knees to pick up the New York Times. He would make himself a cup of coffee and sit down in the blue light of the early morning falling down over the living room. Everything was still as she had left it, the pictures, even the piles of books. Slowly, carefully, he would bend his knees and let himself fall back into the love seat by the window. He would look out onto the park, then slowly he would open the paper, then slowly he would dissolve into it. I watched him the same way I'd watched my mother, standing obscured behind the door. I wanted to see how he really was.

We went out to dinner frequently. We would link arms and walk through the neighborhood to one of our local places. He was trying to fatten up. *I'll order the tempura*, he would say. *I will try to finish it this time.*

He talked about his old age rather professionally. *I've kept your mother's safety bar on the wall of the shower and the plastic chair just so I have it if I need to sit down.* Every day he would do thigh bends against the wall. *There are a couple of moves that are essential to keep your body strong*, he would explain. He applied what he had learned through all his years of work in the field of aging. He spoke of his experience objectively, anecdotally. He wasn't distancing himself from his own pain, but rather, I think, he found his knowledge a great comfort. He understood that everything he faced was a universal truth that everyone faced who survived to a certain age, who outlived their love, who could feel themselves become weakened physically, even mentally as their time grew short. *I am not afraid*, he said, but not to me. He did not like to speak of it to me, as if he felt he was betraying me because I was still young and I needed a father. He wanted to stay. He wanted to meet my child someday, but another part of him was all right with the sense of an approaching end. *I have been lucky in my life*, he said to me. *Work and love have served me well. I have been one of the lucky ones.*

We would sit together in the two La-Z-Boy chairs my mother had bought. He would write by hand. I would type on my laptop. We would read each other passages and offer critiques. We were each working on a book. We left drafts on each other's beds. I would come home to find mine covered in his notes. *Wonderful! Let's discuss at dinner. Meet me in the kitchen 7:30.*

I loved the early evenings in those days, the light seemed as heavy as a fog of red falling over our kitchen. He and I would come home from work. *I could eat Shun Lee,* he'd say. *Or we could go for some thin-crust pizza. I could try to finish one of those.*

We would read the *New York Times* together holding hands.

Do you want a glass of water, Dad? I'm going to get a glass of water.

Sure. And maybe I should have a couple nuts to fatten me up.

The house was quiet. The dog would play and fall asleep on my mother's rug.

Good night, Dad.

Good night, dear. Maybe tomorrow we can get a nice hamburger from that place around the corner. I think I could eat that.

The first night I hung out with Kon we went everywhere, none of which was the kind of place where you might talk about wanting to have babies, or wanting to dress them in a different animal costume each day of the week. But we did. I don't wear heels, but I was wearing three-inch ones that made me four inches taller. He was nonplussed. He smiled up at me, a great wide smile.

I drunkenly babbled that I would adopt a child and raise it by myself, thinking all the while I'd like to throw him on my horse and kidnap him and force him into marriage.

He did not remember me but I remembered him. We'd met before. I knew his name from years ago when he had had his first show at PS 1. The name was unforgettable. Nobody was *Kon.* It sounded like a made-up name, and it turned out it was. He had invented it when he came to the United States from Russia when he was eleven. No one could navigate the name Konstantin at his school in Philly.

I had also seen him at a birthday. He had leaned back woozily through a door to check me out. I was seated in the corner with a friend who was refilling my drink from a flask in her purse. He raised an eyebrow, and I'm sure I turned bright red.

Another time I spotted him seated at a party. I walked over to talk to someone because they were next to him. Unprompted by anything or anyone, he leaned across the table and gave me a very kind smile — *My name is Kon*, he said. *It's nice to meet you.*

I saw him again several months later. A mutual friend began to introduce us but we both finished his sentence. He handed us a bottle of champagne. *I think maybe you two could share this.*

We walked outside. An acquaintance of mine — whom I had liked until he followed us outside — planted himself right between us. After a while we went back in. I was speaking to someone, imagining Kon's eyes on me, but when I turned, he was walking away. I saw the back of his black jacket as he made his way downstairs.

Months later I would ask him about that, and he would say he thought I was too tall to take an interest in him and furthermore — and I think paradoxically — that I was dating my extremely short acquaintance.

Two weeks after we started seeing one another he asked me to marry him, and I actually said yes. It was 4:00 A.M. the day of his birthday. We fell asleep with our shoes on, slept a couple hours, woke, and checked with each other that we meant it.

He came to my father's house to ask for my hand. I hid a tape recorder behind my mother's clock. They spoke about me for twenty minutes then discussed art for three hours. That was basically my father saying yes.

I could sense my mother's happiness when I met Kon, even her wistfulness. This was the man that she had always wanted, but that was not why I was with him. This was the person that I had always wanted. Furthermore, I could not remember what it felt like to not know him. He met my mother through me. He seemed to understand her perfectly.

I told him she had thought too highly of me, that we had been too close, that she had needed to believe that we were special and had chosen each other before birth. I'd believed all her myths, but they had died slowly after her. He said, *Maybe she got some things wrong but she was right about you. I love you as she did. I was born to be your man.*

All good men become great in their old age. My father fell in love with Herta. He was so happy and I was so grateful that for the first time in his life, his focus drifted off his work and onto us—his four daughters and Herta.

He courted her, agonizing over what bracelet he would buy her as a gift. I watched him become the man my mom had always wanted. And though I loved Herta, I felt sad for my mother. At times he had taken her for granted.

I decided love does not always get the time it needs to resolve itself between two people. Yet it does go on resolving in another way as it changes hands. I started to imagine not only my parents as a union but also my mother and Herta as always having been linked.

My mother's death had altered my father. What he learned from losing her made him into a better father, a better man.

When she was sick I sometimes wondered whether my father was a good man. I sometimes wondered if he even loved us. I had expected that he would run off after she died, not want to look at me and see my mother.

I never guessed it would end in the way it did. My father did not run. He clung to me. Finally we could be together without her coming between us. I never would have had that time with him if she had not gone first.

After I met Kon I understood what my father had suffered because I knew the kind of love one shares with a life partner. I hated to imagine Kon ever competing with me over our child. I hated to imagine myself not trusting my own husband or anyone except for my own child.

I knew then that I was not the biggest victim of my mother's loss. I had the world ahead and Kon to start a new life with. But they had been at a certain place of "finally going to." They were finally going to hike Patagonia together. *I might have to carry my old man,* my mother had joked only months before she would fall ill. They were going to stay in a house in

Italy and take afternoon walks together through the vineyards. They were going to write a new kind of book, maybe one of hers for once, maybe her women's history book. They were going to. They were going to.

I failed her, he would say, *amazing Myrna.* Most doctors I know feel that they failed someone in their family. They missed something and that person died, something they might not have missed in a patient. They worry that their judgment was compromised because of their pain.

In my father's case, it was not that he had medically failed my mother but that he had left her alone too long and then in his grief held on to her too long after the point at which she should have been allowed to go. He had focused on saving her until it was too late and he had missed what she really needed from him, which was his help to die, to talk about regrets, about everything.

In his profession, my father had defended as healthy the way older people tend to reminisce, move seamlessly back and forth between the present and the past when they are speaking. He called this "life review," and it became a well-known concept in the field of aging. It went beyond the field. Jane Fonda interviewed my father and later used the term on *Oprah,* though she forgot to give him credit. He had forgotten the importance of his own wife's chance to review her life.

I could not believe that he had run from my mother when she was dying, but of course he ran. She blamed him for her broken dreams. He knew that. He couldn't face her now. They had run out of time. Maybe he blamed himself as much as she blamed him, which would have been too much. Maybe they both could have reached some peace. But my father lacked the courage to risk that they might not.

I learned in those late years with my father that his idea of their story was different from hers. In his mind they were connected but not intertwined.

He had urged her on often to no avail. He found it hard to comprehend her lack of motivation, a lack that comes from a deep-seated belief that you are nothing. This was something he never understood. She had ideas for many different books she never finished. The agreement had been that if she helped Dad with his book *Why Survive?*, he would help her with her books, but it never happened. Like she always said, she should have been given cowriting credit for *Why Survive?*. *My handwriting is all over that manuscript*, she said.

But it took her ten years to write her dissertation, something she saw as a necessity but everybody else knew was just procrastination. During those ten years she would turn to Dad and cry that she couldn't do it, that it was not worth it, that it was not good. When she finally finished her dissertation, her professors urged its publication. She never followed through.

Throughout my life she had tortured herself about the same thing again and again. She had vacillated between thinking she was smarter than my dad and that she was nothing in comparison with him. Either way her game was flawed by the mere position of herself against him. One should not have had to lose for the other to win. Furthermore, she should have kept these thoughts from her child, but she could not, lonely and private as she was, I was the only person she trusted enough. I was imagined by her into some kind of superchild capable of processing her complex emotions. But my simple child's mind computed black and white, and I blamed him, thinking of myself as only her daughter—not his—from an early age.

I began to notice he was napping in the middle of the day. In April, March, in February even, I think he was starting to suspect. His arm started to hurt him. I knew that arm meant something, though doctors seemed to think it was just a shoulder issue.

In July I leaned myself against the thick-paned glass of a roof deck, the top of a hotel staring down into the Hudson River. I noticed that I had missed some calls. They were from my sisters.

Dad told me that I could call you, said Chris.

Kon and I. Elevator down, mirrors on all sides and above. People crowded close together, trying not to linger on their own reflections. It was the second of July.

I had overheard my father speaking to his doctor in March. He said, *No one can explain why I'm losing weight. Myelodysplastic Syndromes, MDS*, she said. *It could develop into leukemia, however at your age, that might never happen. You could just as easily die of something else before that would happen.*

When we arrived at home, my father was halfway off the bed, lying on his back. He asked if I could rub his back with a washcloth.

In the kitchen washing dishes and Chris called. Dad was in the living room where I had left him propped up on the couch with a magazine. The magazine folded in his hand. There were wet spots on the couch from his washcloth he kept pressing to different points along his body as if he were extinguishing small fires.

I told Chris I could not do it again. She told me she would be there tomorrow. I was speaking loudly. Did I want him to hear? I saw it all happening again. We were between the same walls.

He said we should walk out to the park so he would not lose too much strength in his legs. We would go in half an hour, then another, then another. Finally he said he couldn't do it. His robe was slipping, showing his naked body. He strained to lift it as if it were made of stone. I put a blanket over my father.

In the last year of his mother Easter's life, both Dad and I had a hard time. I was eleven and I pushed her away that year, suddenly annoyed by this old woman who had once been my best friend. She was stifling me. I could not stand to spend the time with her I once had spent so easily. She had always needed me so much. When I was little and had friends over for playdates, she would become jealous.

I cannot forget standing over her about six months before she died. She had sunk down onto the floor in the front hallway. My father and I looked down at her. She was sobbing. She took her glasses from her face and threw them across the room.

Get up, Mom, he shouted, *Get up!*

She wailed that she could not, that she was tired. That she just wanted to sit there and to be left alone.

I wanted to kick her I was so angry. I was so afraid.

My father walked away. It was my mother of course who knelt by Easter's side on the floor to comfort her.

Now my father was writing in his bed. I pressed a damp cloth against his skin. He said, *Yes, it helps a little,* and pulled his knees up under his chin. *Take a break,* he kept repeating, *so that you stay sane.*

Tomorrow was the fourth of July. I imagined myself running through a field upstate, where I had planned to be. I recalled sitting in a café with Chris outside the hospital in the early days of my mother's illness. I told Chris that my life was over. She told me I was wrong, that everything would turn out all right. But I felt like I was dying.

This time with my father in the next room I felt the kind of distance I had noticed in my father when my mother was sick. It occurred to me that that distance came out of an accumulation of losses in one's life. There is just so much that you can feel before something inside you adapts. It shuts down the floodlights you felt the first time the pain went burning through your heart.

I started canned soup for him on the stove. We were missing bread. He said he could eat bread. He hadn't had anything all day. I told him I was going to step out, I would be right back. Did he need me to take him to the bathroom?

I walked the couple blocks to the grocery store, then I realized I had not turned off the stove. I started running back. I called him. Could he shut it off? He said he would do it. I was gasping to catch my breath. I phoned him again to tell him to stay put. I saw him crossing the spot where my mother had fallen. I saw his face hitting the stain of blood she'd left. I was pacing in the elevator, cursing. I ran into the hall and flung the door open. There was some black smoke coming from the charred contents of the pot, but there was no fire. I turned the burner off and ran to find my father.

He had made it from the end of his bed to the dresser where she had once fallen. He was stopped, holding on to the dresser. I pulled him into my arms. He felt as light and as tiny as a bird. He rested his forehead on my collarbone.

I'm sorry that I put you through this, Alex.

Don't be sorry, Dad.

Your mother was so worried we would not get along. I think we did quite well.

He died on July 4, a handful of hours after we got to the hospital. Just outside his window fireworks fell down into the Hudson, down over the George Washington Bridge.

New York City summer is always the time when rounding a corner I find myself back in 1982 or 1983. If I don't turn around they are all behind me. My mother, my father, and Grandma Easter.

My childhood happened in the hue of a PBS film about Georgia O'Keefe from 1977 that used to sit on my mother's bookshelf. Sometimes when the light is right I can catch a glimpse of red adobe dust in the concrete.

When I was a little girl I was still too lucky to be lonely. I could love solitude without guilt or fear. Although there were times when a pale sort of feeling would sweep over me, a strange fearful sadness of something yet to come. In the playground I watched other children, was for years uncertain how to lose myself in their play.

This July is hot. I lie behind the drawn shade of my father's window. The house harks back, teases me it could slip out of today into another better one sometime before. And as I look back I realize some of my best days in my life were with my father in the last years of his. Even though at the time I was completely lost, twenty-seven, no career, no relationship, and worst of all, no plan, completely uncertain.

But the fact that I had lost my mom allowed me to be happy. I knew to lose myself in being with my dad.

Please let me stay home, he had said when Chris told him go to the Palliative Care Unit. I think he knew he would not return.

The next time I saw him blue plastic framed the edges of his face. It stuck out of the hole cut in the paper he was wrapped in. He had been autopsied. Blue plastic kept the sheets he lay in dry.

Cindy touched his face. I did not want to know how he felt cold. Over the last two years if he fell asleep, I would stare at him. I would imagine him dead. It helped me remember what was left to say. I would wake him as I had so many times longed to wake my mother.

Now he was swaddled, still white, and this was real. And I realized I had forgotten to make him promise me he would say good-bye. He snuck away just as he had done with my mom.

There was a voice message from three weeks before, but I erased that. That was strange. I was prone to save such things. His messages were letters read aloud, and they always ended *Love, Dad*. I wrote down what I could remember.

Dear Alex,

I watch you beat yourself up that you have not accomplished enough with your life. You took care of your mother. You wrote your first book. You learned another language. You got a master's degree. You found a best friend to spend your life with. I think that if you sat on your duff for the rest of your days, you would have done enough.

When he died, the doctor told me everything, but her words were a foreign language, a series of sounds strung together with no space. I came home with my father's clothes folded in my hands. I spent a week sitting at my computer doing searches on his name, and on his illness.

Damaged blood-producing cells in bone marrow—trouble making new cells—low numbers of one or more type cells.

"Dr. Robert N. Butler, a psychiatrist whose painful youthful realization that death is inevitable prompted him to challenge and ultimately reform the treatment of the elderly through research, public policy, and a Pulitzer Prize–winning book . . ."

Blood cells made by damaged cells are not normal—body will destroy them.

"He worked until three days before his death . . . acute leukemia."

Blast crisis—increase in proportion of blast cells—fever or pain in bones. Symptoms might include joint pain. Patient may be asymptomatic or have mild symptoms of fatigue.

"Dr. Butler's influence was apparent in the widely used word he coined, 'ageism.' He defended as healthy the way many old people slip into old memories—even giving it a name, 'life review.'"

Blast crisis is the final phase.

"... *Dr. Butler had in effect 'created an entire field of medicine.'*"

For the first time I wanted to keep him held in the context of who he'd been in the larger world. I started watching his and my mother's old TV interviews. I wanted to push the fire he described burning through his body away and see him in those old 1970s suits, that terrible side part and my mother in that old pageboy haircut. I didn't want to think about when Kon and I first found him halfway off his bed, his palms pressed on the floor. We pulled him up, his hands curling as if they were deep-fried and his teeth grinding down into his lip.

Light as a child in my arms he was when I helped him to the bathroom, this father who hoisted me once onto his shoulder. His doctors called twice a day from their weekends away for the Fourth of July. He wanted to stay at home until their return. He did not trust the care of strangers.

He said he was better off at home. *Too much illness at the hospital*, he said.

Summer storms and fireworks and both of them were taken in July.

I'm sorry, he and I kept saying in that fury of last days because we both knew how these things go. We stared into each other's eyes, feeling that familiar void work its way up between us.

When my father was four years old he looked up from playing in the yard and saw a strange man standing by the fence. He knew it was his father. He began to cry and ran into the house. That was the last time my father ever saw his dad.

My father always described his childhood in a Huckleberry Finn way, but after he died when I think of those stories without the inflection of his voice, the genre is no longer the same. I picture him young on a wooden bench in a courtroom watching his grandmother beg to keep their house despite their debt and losing it. I see him abandoned by his father, abandoned by his mother, abandoned when his grandfather dies.

When my mom became sick, I had seen him as the lucky one, the one with choices, the one who was not generous enough to stay by her side. I never considered that no one had ever taught him how to say good-bye.

All the month of June he had searched the house for a book he had had since childhood. It was a book of two-minute biographies of over twenty different people—writers, scientists, and so on. He never found it.

How many abandoned children are left to model their lives on a such a book? There were many times when I felt his narrow flashlight of a focus leave me in the black, lock me outside those biography pages he longed to complete and secretly hoped someday his father would read.

He had always spoken of his father with indifference, saying his grandpa was enough. He had spoken of his mother taking off with humor. She was like a sister who would sweep through town, beautiful and kind, then be on her way. He made his childhood sound so breezy, so different from the way my mother described hers. I took that at face value. But going through his papers, I saw that he had searched for his father at one point and discovered his father was dead.

The dead behave differently than when they were alive. I watch my father like a film reel. I see everything another way. He read every one of his favorite books in those last months, *War and Peace*, anything written by Camus. He kept saying to me, *Let's pick the place where we will hold your wedding.* Chris told me that in February he said he was satisfied. He said he hoped he could walk me down the aisle, to hold my first child but indicated that he thought that was ambitious.

I had worried over the wrong thing and missed what was unfolding. It was the final hours of his life. And I was pacing myself, keeping myself remote so as not to make the same mistake I had with her, so as not to become exhausted.

On the last day of his life he kept demanding more pain medication. I hadn't slept, and all I wanted was quiet on a chair in the corner of the room for just a minute. I kept telling him to wait a bit, that the medication would kick in. That was the last time that we spoke. It never occurred to me that he was demanding the first of his last dose, the one that would knock him from consciousness. He had no intention of coming home.

I spent days going through my parents' things. I spent nights in their bed with my head pressed into my father's pillow. My dreams were the only funny thing about my life, comically literal dreams of my father. In these dreams he never showed himself, but I always knew he was close by.

In one dream he hid behind an elephant leaf my aunt had included in a poem about him. It was giant and electric green. I asked him to show himself. He would not, but I could see his shoes shiny and black that he had been buried in.

I pulled everything out of their closets, yanked all the boxes off the shelves. My parents did not throw much away. All throughout my childhood there were piles and piles of papers, books, and things around the house. It drove me crazy. They would get so angry at me when they came home to find I had hidden them away, even when I was five, stuffed them all into drawers and out of sight. Clutter was never something I could bear, and less so now.

Each day several new business cards of "estate salesmen" would appear in the mail pile. I called one of the numbers. A man's voice—he said he'd come today. I pulled out the folding tables from my mother's closet that she kept for parties or for doing taxes. I went around the house picking things up and spread them on the tables. My sisters and I had already claimed the things we wanted. The handful of items of real value that my parents owned had been appraised and set aside. This was all the rest, the tchotchkes, the costume jewelry, the strange cuff links from my father's drawer, the hideous ties he never wore. Each item looked up at me through orphan eyes. I whispered to myself, *These things are not your parents*.

I eyeballed the items on the tables as if walking through a street fair. I made a little pile of things I'd decided last-minute to keep. I sat down and waited on the man. I got up and added some things to my pile. I got up and took some things away. The doorbell sounded.

The man looked like he was out of central casting. Four strands of greasy hair thin as veins stretched over his scalp. Dry lips, liver spots, and Coke-bottle glasses like my mother's that made his eyes incredibly small. He wore dirty-looking high-waist polyester pants, had multiple pens shoved in his chest pocket. The elevator lingered open after he stepped out. The others inside seemed to be asking me if I really wanted this guy to come in.

Dabbing at his nose with a yellowed handkerchief, he inquired if he could use my bathroom. I almost said no. Emily growled. I told myself I'd deluge that bathroom with some Clorox when he left.

We commenced our business at the first table.

I'll give you five.

I won't take less than eight.

I felt like I was at the Gypsy market in Seville, Spain, where at eighteen I had had to buy my own bike back at a heightened price. Except this time I was the Gypsy. He pressed crunchy new bills into my hand. I counted them up and shoved them deep into the tote bag that was hanging from my shoulder.

That day I would sell my mother's silver, the set that she loved and I hated with the flowers on the handle. I would get $19,000 in cash for various belongings. I wanted him to take it all, take it for free. I wished all the walls would fade to white. I wished for the house to become empty either by flood or fire.

I tore through the things he wouldn't take, threw them into boxes I stacked by the door. I broke the paper shredder feeding it too fast—twenty-year-old receipts, old yellowed letters from dead friends to my parents. The ones I saved I put in a box for my father's secretary to go through and gauge whether to keep them for posterity.

They had kept files on every trip they'd ever taken. *Vain, vain, vain,* I clucked away, crumpling brochures from hotels populated by figures in

1980s clothing, 1970s clothing—1960s clothing, for Christ's sake. I filled bag after bag with these papers.

I came across my mother's files on me, worthy of the Stasi in their nearly minute-by-minute accounting. She had even assumed other identities at times. She had a "friend" when I was little, a Mrs. McGillicuddy, who tended to come around when I had tantrums.

My mother would leave the room and then I'd hear a knock.

Is Alexandra there? a southern voice would trill.

Yes, I would say at two, three, and four years old.

I knew it was my mother and yet it was another iteration. This southern lady was someone new I could talk to. Someone who was not wearing my mother's frustrated expression. She was calm. She came from a better place. She always came with teacups in her hand. We would sit down cross-legged on the floor, eye to eye, to discuss the inner workings of my childhood mind. My face might still be red or wet with tears, but I would tell her calmly the reason that I was having a tantrum.

What might I suggest to your mother that she do to help ferry you out of this squall? Mrs. McGillicuddy always asked the same question last so often I would have my answer ready before she even knocked. I would give an answer, and after some business like back and forth we would adjourn. *I'll go find your mother then.* And off Mrs. McGillicuddy went.

Other times she and I would wrestle on the living room floor. My dad would play the role of referee—there were no hits to the face, there were no hits at all, only our interpretations of classic wrestling moves. Remembering these moments, I would laugh out loud in my parents' house, stop what I was doing, and see them smile at me through a thin veil inches from my face, and I would smile back.

I continued with my mother's files on me. She had kept her favorites of my childhood drawings organized by year. I looked at each one. I was good. I was really good. I just didn't get better. At twelve I was making the same crap I had made at five.

I saved several and crumpled the rest. I could hear her gasping, having saved all of this for me. For me to do what? Maybe she thought someday she would sit down with this stuff and reminisce—that "someday" come and gone. I tore up all the drawings. I tore up the white cardboard boxes they had been held in. I recycled it all.

I found the boxes of my baby clothes that she had kept, a label with my name sewn into each and every one. There were baby-size feminist T-shirts that proclaimed a woman's right to choose. I kept those, of course. There were orange polyester baby bell-bottoms. I kept those as well because they were so ugly no one would believe me unless I kept them as proof.

I went through maybe a thousand books, kept about two hundred, and donated the rest except those whose pages came apart in my hands. I dropped three closets' worth of clothes at the Housing Works donation desk.

After the books, the papers, all the contents of the house had met their day, I went for the Big Five—the furniture, rugs, exercise equipment, wall units, and electronics.

At midnight, 1:00 A.M., 2:00 A.M., I hauled furniture I swear I could not carry today. I lined all of it up by the back door as far away from me as I could get it short of putting it outside. I hired two gentlemen who worked in the building to pick these items up and drive them off in a big truck, I did not know to where.

I jumped up and down on her wooden bed tray. It was coming apart anyway. I ripped her safety bar right off the shower wall. I let the twenty-five-year-old television I had watched cartoons on as a child drop from my hands.

This left the piano. When I was two she began to sit me down in front of the piano. My legs straight out in front of me couldn't clear the bench. She would slide me right up to edge and hold me by the waist so that I wouldn't fall. Sometimes she would tape-record the vile rackets I made. From three to thirteen I practiced almost every day. I staunchly believe that it is the only reason I'm able to concentrate. It combated the mind decimation of TV. I can see her fingers drumming on the side of the piano, her glasses traveling back and forth from her face to the page.

She considered my fits as simply a part of the process. Together we hurricaned through each developmental phase, making the best music we could manage. I thought at the time that it was I who suffered, but now I understand it must have been a hell for her. I was not an easy child if I did not want to be. I moaned, as if in utter agony, into the keys of the piano. I lay beneath its belly collapsed on the floor howling as if I were a dying dog. In moments like this she would drown my sound out by playing an Art Landry tune from 1925. *Five foot two, eyes of blue . . . Has anybody seen my girl?* I would gaze from my point of death at her foot thumping at the pedal in tune to the demonic tick of the metronome.

At four I had a new teacher, a straight-backed ballerina who taught out of her five-hundred-square-foot apartment. There was no furniture, only Persian rugs. Just two grand pianos lined up as bride and groom and three uprights pushed against a wall.

She always wore her hair one of three ways: a tight, high bun, some conglomeration of braids, or down and wild in her eyes. Some days she wore ribbons like a little girl. I found this as a child to be shocking. Some days she was made up like a Russian doll with red lips and white powder. Other days she looked like she'd been up playing piano like a wild woman since dawn. I was too young to realize she was my first artist. When I was five she started me on the recital circuit. Of course my mother had found her.

When I was battling daily with my mother before, on top of, or beneath her piano, my father would go slinking past the door afraid to be recruited in some way. We were beyond his helpless reach. But at their dinner parties I would play Bach, Beethoven, and Stravinsky in my tiny party dress. And then my father would begin to gasconade about the vital nature of childhood music training. She would roll her eyes and squeeze my hand under the table. Sometimes my dad noticed us giggling at him—our little clique was already in full swing. It is hard to say what kind of father my dad would have been had she not been around. I will never know.

I sold the piano to a man who came and lovingly gazed at it a while and played it well enough. I needed the money. I needed to unload the weight of that piano more.

At night Kon would come from the studio and I'd be like a hamster tearing everything around me into shreds. He joked that I had gotten started on my mother's steroids. This prompted a visit to the medicine cabinet, where we selected my father's painkillers, the ones he took on the last day of his life. We lay down on the bed, held hands, and watched TV and let ourselves slowly go to Jell-O.

hi this is dad are you getting this

I wake up in tears, having converted Cindy's story of teaching our father how to text into a dream. Kon said all the right things, that he would never leave me; that he had loved my father; that he would always keep my father with him; that my father was the best man he had ever known; that he had promised my father he would take care of me. And as much as I loved Kon in that moment, I could feel myself being pulled by my ankles down into my own throat, down into the blackness of my chest.

There were piles of things that I saved for last, her lace that she loved so much—I couldn't stand to see it anymore. There was still some furniture I couldn't throw away. Kon's mother offered to take it. She would keep it at her house upstate until I knew what to do with it. I hired a moving company and piled it back to back down in her basement. This is the only reason I rock my baby in the same chair I was rocked in.

I promised myself I would never live or die with more sheets in the closet than I used. I photographed some of the things I had thrown away— over three hundred pictures on my phone that later that year would accidentally be erased.

On the day the painters came, I sat at the kitchen table. I felt a memory rise up around me. I felt my favorite nightgown against my skin, white and covered with red berries. The phone rings, my father answers. It is Easter.

Maybe she says, *Neil* [my father's middle name], *how is Alexandra?*

Maybe he says, *She is eating her daddy's famous succotash.*

I smile and show him the contents of my mouth.

Does she want me to sleep over?

I nod my head vehemently and roar like a lion, *Yes! Yes! Yes!*

I think you heard that, Ma, my father says.

It is six o'clock, my old dinnertime. Easter will arrive and read me to sleep from the rocking chair. She will drift off, and I will chuck a teddy at her shins to wake her up. And like a little engine revving and powering the sentence that was lost in the middle, she is back.

Take the table home, I say to one of the painters. *It's too heavy for me to deal with.* Three and a half weeks after I started, my family's house was empty. On that sunny Sunday morning I walked from the building, Emily pulled me forward on her leash. We passed my parents' bench with their names engraved onto the plaque. A little more than one year before I saw my father there snoozing in the sun. I was late to an appointment, but I stopped to sit with him. And I remember thinking, *This is a feeling you'll remember, the sun on your face and your father's hand in yours.* I remember knowing that I would be so glad to arrive quite late to that appointment.

This Sunday morning I let Emily off her leash and watched her run into the green, bellowing as if she were a child. I remember blossoms falling, although it was too late in the year. I stood in the center of the field watching her run. A man leaning against the rocks began to play the bandoneon. Then and there he played my parent's favorite song, "Adiós Nonino."

Kon and I moved into a place downtown. We painted it. We made it a home. Our neighbor had long stringy black hair and he would shout and grunt every time he climbed the six-floor walk-up. As soon as he closed his apartment door behind him he would scream as if releasing what he had had to hide out in the world.

I understood that I was sad. The type of sad that compels you to live in the moment. I thought I had my head right. I didn't have my head right. I became convinced the bathroom mirror was double sided, that my neighbor was watching.

Late at night I could hear him drilling, and I worried he was slowly building a passageway through the wall to us. I heard him scratching on the walls. I would awaken Kon and clamp my hand over his mouth. I would get up in the middle of the night, half asleep, to check the lock of the front door. I looked through the keyhole to make sure he wasn't there each time I left. I worried that he would push poison through the crack of our front door and kill Emily. I would lock her in the bedroom every time I left the house.

Every Sunday when I was very small, my mother would make a little breakfast and put it on a tray. She used a little Russian tea set, and each plate held its little something. I was not allowed to eat on the carpet in front of the TV, so she would park me just outside the door. I would watch *The Smurfs*. She would disappear into my room.

I think a little elf came, she would say taking my hand. My bedroom would be spotless, my bed made, all the toys put away. My gerbil, Brendan, would be running in ecstatic laps the length of his freshly scrubbed cage. This was the first phase of my mother's turning me into a neat freak. This was how she created the need inside me.

When I turned four she started a new thing called Major Cleanups. She would put me in charge of finding all the books around my room and putting them together in a group. When I had done that, she would give me another category—dolls or cars or maybe records.

In our new apartment downtown I cleaned all the time to calm myself. I was angry with my father for dying in the middle of summer. That left me fall and winter to get through. And it was as early as October when the pain started in my stomach and back.

I watched videos of Dad on the Internet. I read interviews that he had done. I cut my hair. Then cut my hair again until it was only an inch long. I went through the two boxes I had brought down from his house, his chicken scratch on envelopes, his notes on the memoir that he could not write. On the back of a Post-it note I read, *The importance of dreaming.* It occurred to me I wasn't dreaming. Kon and I had to plan our wedding in ten months, now nine months, now eight.

Kon would give me assignments that I would muddle through. Soon he was planning it alone. He said he liked to do it. I knew that that was partly true, but he was being kind. *I want to marry you,* I would say, grasping his shoulders. *I want to marry you.* And I did. I just could not care about the tablecloths or silverware. It hurt him I think because he felt I was floating away. I *was* floating away and would have disappeared if I did not love him so much.

I moved through the day like a wild dog wearing a woman's clothing, hiding underneath a veil of disguise. I should have come home with broken nails on my feet and hands, with gravel on my face from dragging and writhing around. My friends told me often I seemed well considering. Did they leave a pause for me to fill? Did they give me an opening? There was no opening big enough for what I had to say. So I stayed silent. Or I would put forth curated words I felt hung well together in a crosslike shape around my neck. I wanted to be attractive enough that I would not be abandoned. I could not stand one more ounce of solitude.

I felt myself disappear anytime Kon was not in front of me, like an infant that cannot conceive of what is not in front of its face. He would come home and I would jump into his arms, pull him down onto the bed, eye to eye. My mother wrote in my baby book, *She loves to put her face close to me and speak from the heart even though she does not use words.* These months are barren landscapes or they are Kon's face eye to eye, his hands in mine, his smile. I would jump out of myself then and into us. My body filled with blood again, my organs, my bones came back to life. This is perhaps the only reason I survived.

As winter carried on the pain grew worse. I slowly realized that I was now in the middle of the meat. I was the meat. The pain was expanding, a separate being feeding on me now. It laughs. I am the joke. I read that Gershwin died at thirty-eight of a brain tumor. How was that not the first thing anyone ever said about Gershwin?

I called my doctor and begged for an appointment the same day. I asked for blood tests. I saw a chiropractor, who explained in great detail what I had going on. I have since forgotten what he called it, but he said there was something in my stomach that was popping out of place. I was prepared to believe anything—try anything. I saw him twice a week. I would feel relief a couple days and then it would come back.

I lay down in the middle of the day. I made space for the pain in my life. Slowly I forgot that it was strange. Maybe everyone had pain like this, maybe this wasn't even pain. Maybe it was life.

At our wedding he was waiting by the altar. All the year before he had gently pulled me toward the day. I had no doubt that I wanted to marry him. Not one doubt, and yet all I could think was that this shaman friend of my sister's had said he heard my parents in the trees. They were behind us in the trees. I did not feel sad about that or comforted or even as if I understood that as meaning anything at all. I also did not feel the happiness and joy I thought that I should feel. Even when I looked into his face and felt such relief and gratitude that he was still there despite the fact that I was barely there or anywhere, even then I still felt nothing. I was as light and transparent as each layer of cloth that made up my wedding dress. So I tried to draw myself together, keep myself together as the layers on that dress that combined made it opaque enough to keep safe what was inside.

I arrived at my wedding late, around the time they carried Kon and me high up on chairs. That was the moment I was married, one year to the day of my father's death. We set off fireworks. I told myself dancing in Kon's arms that this day would mark the ending of my grief. The first night of our honeymoon we were exhausted from the wedding. I put my head on the restaurant table as a joke. And then I fell asleep. We had come to the Berkshires, empty tomato soup cans tied to our car. I surprised myself saying I wanted to get pregnant. Kon smiled. Neither one of us said it but we both knew I wasn't well enough.

Early the next morning my mother came to me in a dream holding a baby. The baby was a dummy made of wood, a ventriloquist's doll. I woke up angry. Kon found me crying as he would find me many times that year.

With my father's death I felt as if I'd lost her again. The first year, they were these two wraiths standing before me and blocking my view almost to the point of blindness. I imagined—I dreamed—whatever it was I spent all that year doing—my mother as transparent, my father as opaque. She had let a great deal of her connection to me go. He could not. Or maybe it was I who could not. I felt we were one another's captives. We had found our love too late. And lost it too soon. At first it had seemed right to imagine her as free, and imagine my father as regretful. Yet the more I stared into the memory of them, the more their identities started to unravel.

He still had the presence of a house cat, curled up on every chair. I felt certain he had been his truest self the last years of his life. And that made me long for the years that I had missed of being close to him. Years where he could have influenced me, influenced who I would become.

I realized how closed off I had always been to my father. As far back as I had memory I had believed he had nothing to offer. It had never occurred to me that I was just as much his child as hers, just as likely to inherit his traits as to inherit hers. Yet she had made me believe I was a facsimile of her.

Now I understood for the first time how much I had in common with my father, this man who had been described by my mother as alien to her and me. If she had let me be, I might have been like him, might have been better. I began to look back at different periods of my life and imagine them improved by my turning to him instead of always to her. She had stolen him from me.

I uncovered memories that would become well worn over that year. I thought about his sunniness, how he could be merry on the surface even when he was suffering. I remembered rituals I had not always perceived as rituals, the fact that he would sit me on the sink when I was small so I could help him shave.

The Nantucket Reds war was six years long over a pair of salmon shorts. These shorts were a gift from a friend my father stayed with in Nantucket. *Now you are a local,* he had said. My father loved that sort of talk. But he was not a local, not even when he was at home. He was a nerd from another planet wearing a beret in Paris that read "Paris." My mother hated those Nantucket Reds, but when she dropped them in the trash, he would pull them out.

There were the endless rounds of tickle monster that we played, chasing one another through the house. He would come prancing toward me, lifting his knees high, jutting his chin out, and baring his teeth, the cartoon villain.

I would go with him to get his hair cut on 113th Street by Columbia from a lady named Ricky. In our swivel chairs beaming at each other, Dad would rave to me about how Ricky was *the greatest barber in the world.* Not hyperbole, he truly believed that about well over half the people he knew. He considered it simply good luck that he seemed to meet the most talented people in the world. I realized the good luck was his good humor and that the way he saw the world was the way he made it.

I remembered his impersonations and his characters that he invented through the years. There was Squeako the Pig with a voice you can imagine.

I recalled how he and I used to tape the show *That's Entertainment,* practice the dance moves, and invent routines. I danced on his feet so he would not step on mine.

He was my encyclopedia. I left questions on scrap paper outside his bedroom door. He left answers on scrap paper outside mine. I loved his answers, balanced and cool and quite close to objective. I believed in the world from his perspective.

He was constantly working, and yet if I needed him, it required a simple tug of his sleeve. He would drop everything and give me his full attention. He was so happily pulled out of concentrated work and just as easily reabsorbed. He could work in a place pulsing with life. He could breeze in and out of the fray. His work and life were seamlessly interconnected. He never took a day completely off. This drove my mother crazy, but not, I think, for the reason she said. I think it drove her crazy because she longed to be the same.

That year he came to me in little motion pictures that could pull me out of wherever I was. There he was padding around our apartment on a Sunday, wearing one in a rotating line of kimonos from a Japanese airline's business class. He would spend hours in his chair, one leg crossed over the other, his glasses on a cord around his neck getting tangled in his shirt. He is so deep in a book only his ears are visible; a half-eaten package of saltines is on his lap.

Later on he will be in the kitchen by the phone trying to decide between Shun Lee and his homemade spaghetti. He will burn the spaghetti and set off the smoke detector, which he'll take down from the ceiling before cracking the window to get rid of the smoke.

Sometimes I can almost hear his voice. That vocal spectrum that could range from booming to falsetto and hit both extremes inside one sentence. He was funny. There was not one suit in the entire world that fit that man, those narrow, sloping shoulders, the barrel chest, the knock-kneed legs. And yet he was dashing, one of the most handsome fathers in the world.

I would watch him on TV in an interview, one pant leg ridden up, exposing a kneesock that, having aborted its mission. now clung midcalf and clumped about his ankle. There was not a speck of concern about judgment or rejection. He was always certain the world would love him back.

That was why she had been so mad at him. She wanted that. We all deserve that. He ate life in big triumphant gulps, while she merely nibbled at the edge of some giant dreams she never did go for.

She had always taken credit for bringing the family together after her intrusion. Now that did not seem as real to me after watching everybody shuffle during her illness, after her death, after Dad's death. Cindy once said when we were fighting over our father's love long after he had died, *I could have hated you but I didn't. You were my first child. Our relationship is indefinable. I feel so many things for you that I can't even explain them, but the greatest one is love.*

I realized everyone had fought and sacrificed, everyone had worked just as hard as my mother.

Dad once described my mother as having *a bell in her voice*. I don't know if he pulled that from a book. Why did that bell not ring for me anymore? Why could I turn only to my father now that they were both gone? My need for him was so profound, more profound even than I had ever had for her. Because it was the ache of a parent lost long before he was found and then lost again.

Douglas Martin wrote the following of my father in the *New York Times*, July 7, 2010:

His parents had scarcely named him Robert Neil Butler before splitting up 11 months after his birth. . . . He went to live with his maternal grandparents on a chicken farm in Vineland, N.J. He came to revere his grandfather, with whom he cared for sick chickens in the "hospital" at one end of the chicken house. He loved the old man's stories. But the grandfather disappeared when Robert was 7, and nobody would tell him why. . . . Robert found solace in his friendship with a physician he identified only as Dr. Rose. Rose helped him through scarlet fever and took him on his rounds by horse and carriage. The boy decided he could have helped his grandfather survive had he been a doctor. He concluded that he would have preferred that people had been honest with him about death. From his grandmother, he learned about the strength and endurance of the elderly. . . . After losing the farm in the Depression, she and her grandson lived on government surplus foods in a cheap hotel. Robert sold newspapers. Then the hotel burned down, with all their possessions. "What I remember even more than the hardships of those years was my grandmother's triumphant spirit and determination," he wrote. "Experiencing at first hand an older person's struggle to survive, I was myself helped to survive as well." . . . Dr. Butler acknowledged in an interview two years ago with the *Saturday Evening Post* that his views on his own aging had changed; he feared death less. "I feel less threatened by the end of life than I perhaps did when I was 35," he said.

I used to tell myself that I was lucky. The ones who run suffer the most. I didn't run, not when she was sick, not when he was sick. So I should feel complete. I should feel I did the best I could, that I didn't run. But I don't feel resolved. Resolved about their deaths maybe, not about their lives.

When she was dying, I perceived the distance as coming from my father, but she and I were pushing him away. I realize now I wanted him to fail. She had set us up to compete. The three of us never cried together. My father and I passed my sick mother back and forth as if we had never learned to share her.

Maybe some things were too painful not to throw out at the start. He was avoiding what he knew lay between them all those years. He had run out of time to fix what she told him needed fixing. But he was not responsible for her unhappiness. Some martyrs self-select as martyrs and leave as victims all those whom they put before themselves. He did not always do right by her. He was selfish, he was sexist—all of that. But she also did not do right by him. Most of all she was terrible to herself. She never understood that she would have to stop that to be happy and go after what she really wanted.

Now I had this memory of him. Several months before my father died, he asked if I would come with him. The vet was putting his cat, Charlotte, down. She had been my mother's pet, and when my mother died, she began to sleep on her pillow. She would spend all night sleeping next to my dad. He put his face down on the table so he was eye to eye with her. *Charlotte, you have been a good cat.* Her white paws lay one over the other, graceful as ballet slippers, and he held them in his hand as she died.

In the fall after my wedding, I started to find marks all over my body. I would start to choke when I drank, knock things over all the time. I started to have cramps in my pelvis and my groin. My left breast felt as if it were on fire. Both my wrists were sore. The nerves up and down my arm felt pinched, and I felt as if I had an invisible string tied around my thumb. There seemed to be something pressing on my spine, and my pelvis was popping out of place, my coccyx left to right. There was a painful spot above my belly button, as if I'd been sliced open. I was sore down both sides of my neck. My ankles felt jammed into my feet, and my knees pulsed with ache. I had this clicking in my breastbone and cracks and pops inside my chest. There was this vibrating chord of pain along both sides of my waist. My feet engorged during long sits, turned blue and purple-brown. I couldn't concentrate, couldn't spell, was photosensitive, flipped my letters upside down. My muscle tone decreased, my belly distended. I was diagnosed with Lyme disease.

I would travel up to Sinai and see my father's cohorts, old men now, gentleman doctors you no longer find. They all seemed to know my father or know of him. They shared their memories with me. I would lie on the examination table and just close my eyes. I was diagnosed with fibromyalgia. I was rapidly losing weight. One young doctor covering one day informed me that I might have cancer.

I went home to Kon. I went crying, and yet there was a real glimmer of hope that I would be going to them. Kon would lie down on the bed with me, but when he put his hands on me, I just flew away. We were one year into marriage and he said, *I will not leave you. Not even in ten years if you're this way. Even though I should.*

That was the worst time, when I did not know what was wrong with me and I wanted nothing. I could not see who I was without my parents. I could not rally and I could not rest. Falling to sleep or waking, I would touch exquisite pain and understand what it was I carried in my heart even though I could not feel it. I was living like a rhesus monkey clinging to a mother made of wire. My eyes were turned inward ransacking the chamber of my grief for anything of value.

Kon started to beg me to come back as if I weren't next to him. His tone started to become panicked. He promised I would never be alone. But I had been promised this before. As long as he and I lived in separate bodies, we would always be alone, we would always be at risk of losing one another. He was so innocent, though. He had that naïveté that death takes. He said, *If you reject the world, eventually it will drift away.* He said, *Don't wait too long to join me here.*

After more tests and more consultations with doctors, we would come to understand I did not have Lyme disease or fibromyalgia or cancer. I had depression. I was put on Zoloft. I would call my doctor every day asking when the pain would end.

Kon and I were in Los Angeles at the time for a show he had of paintings. We house-swapped with a friend who lived in a house in Echo Park.

I knew the house was beautiful, but I couldn't quite enjoy it or anything else. The pain was going but so also was feeling—emotions seemed to elude me. I spent my first days sitting on the back porch in the sun wondering if it would erase me.

Every day my friend Andrea would appear at the door and take me walking slowly through the canyons. Kon was at the gallery finishing the show, and he would step outside to call me every couple of hours. The first two weeks passed this way, and then I started to feel normal.

When I was young I used to build cities. I never tired of it, pulling my parents' objects down, their knickknacks and coasters, inventing stories. Now I felt I could do that again.

I found a letter from Irene folded up in the back of a journal my mother kept about my birth.

Dear Myrna,

These are our inner feelings for our 12th grandchild. Father, after many years of waiting You have given us our lovely granddaughter Alexandra Nicole and we thank You with our whole heart. What a miracle! Those features of the face with the little nose and mouth, the eyes and ears, the beautiful hands, the perfect feet and toes. Lord, I will praise Thee for I am fearfully and wonderfully made, marvelous are Thy works and that my soul knows right well. Lord, we pray, that as parents Your love, patience, wisdom, and firmness will give Myrna the ability to be a good example to Alexandra but above all give her the kind of love that is reflective of Your divine love. May You always consider Alexandra to be a precious gift from You. And Father, keep her safe in Your care, we ask this in Jesus' name. And please God let no harm come to the parents and Alexandra. With love to all Thine . . .

Mother and Dad

I reach into what separates my mother and me and pull her back to me fiber by fiber, molecule by molecule. I understand the why of everything she was. In her death, I have beaten her up. I have dragged her good name through the dirt. I had to do it, had to pluck her from the tree and throw her on the ground, but she returned, more beautiful, more real. She gave me the language to take her down and take her apart. Most important, she gave me the certainty that she would understand, that she would forgive me—even cheer me on. She avoided her biggest fear, which I think was that I could have a life, a mother like that letter, so distant, so disconnected.

As I write about her I know my mother is always behind me. After all it was she who taught me how to write. She was a loving tyrant, a cockeyed conductor, red pen in her hand over my head. She was tough. I had to revise my third grade report on Turkey eleven times. I remember lying under the computer table curled up like a kicked dog staring at her red snakeskin heels. *The jig is up,* she said. *When you finish your fit, we'll go on to page two.* Her hand came down to give me a pat. I batted it away. On that black IBM screen with the ghostly green text my sentences were halved then halved again. *Each thought must be completed but not over-stated in order to move on.* This was not advice only for writing.

The contradictions I saw in them, in their lives, their illness, death, hung me up a while. I was tormented by the idea that they were not the people I had believed them to be.

But now I understand that few things are more human than consistent contradiction. That we all in some way will fail the ones we love. We all lie to ourselves and to each other, at times unbeknownst to us, at times consciously in order to survive. It is hard for me to say whether all I have written is true, what it was I lived and what I imagined. This is fine. If you want them to, the dead come back and you can continue on with them. You can build them back into your life

There were times I hated my father when she was dying. Now his weakness soothes me. His imperfection was the greatest gift that he ever gave me.

The life that I shared with them has returned. For years I could feel only the sadness and the terror of their end. But they left a time capsule in me, and one day it was opened. Then the innocence and joy of the life I shared with them seemed real again. Real as the hardship and the horror that took them.

I had let them go. I was two months pregnant, standing in a restaurant, and I saw a woman dazed, black eyed, with navy-blue bruises down her face. She dragged one leg behind her like an axe. Her husband, frail as she, walked alongside, and I could not tell who was leaning on whom. I cried but I didn't stay. I walked home with the feeling that I was accompanied again in that way that happens only between a mother and child.

All I know now is I am grateful, grateful for exactly who they were, for everything unfolding as it did, for the mistakes I no longer call mistakes, and the betrayals I no longer call betrayals. I am happy for their deaths exactly as they happened.

They shone as two people so much and adored me so much; I never felt that I had earned it. I never felt their love was truly reflective of me. It was all theirs. They would have given it to any child born to them. I had to fight to love myself. I had to feel that I had struggled, that I had earned my value through crawling up from pain. Earning my own love is better than having theirs or anybody else's. Yet the ability to understand how to love myself—it comes from them; another contradiction.

Down in the center of my suffering, in the raw middle of the meat, I found a self I did not know. This self knew her way in war and was a mother, long before she had one. Once the pain had stopped, I found it a relief to be nobody's child. I had finally come home.

All I know is this: My mother was wrong about herself and her life. She shone throughout her life. But her functioning was a performance to mask the terrified woman behind. Instead of declaring war on that insecurity, she declared war alternatively on my father, on the world, on herself. It would have been more painful for her to realize that she had been holding herself back than to tell herself that she was oppressed and that the things she felt deprived of never could have been hers. The life she could have had but did not fight for was too painful to conceptualize.

All I know is this: I was born to Bob and Myrna in a golden time. And they gave me credit for it. We lived in a tree house on the Upper West Side. The potted plants in the living room were thick as a forest. Their leaves tapped the windows that opened on the blue. Our days were lush as drawings dripping from a page. We loved one another. We were lucky.